THE
AUTOIMMUNE
PROTOCOL
REINTRODUCTION
COOKBOOK

Nourishing Recipes for Every Stage of Your Healing Journey

FAIR WINDS

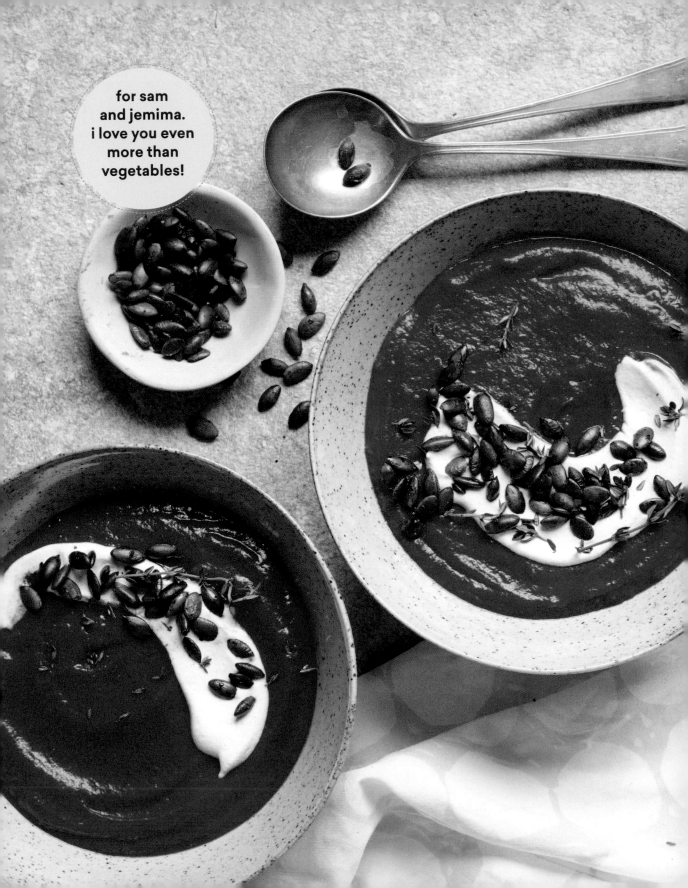

for sam and jemima. i love you even more than vegetables!

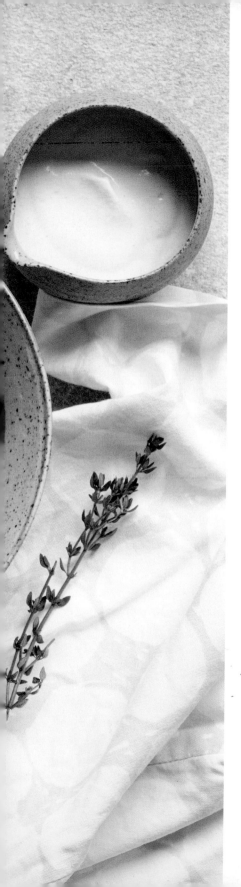

CONTENTS

FOREWORD

I HAD ALREADY BEEN living with the autoimmune illness, lichen planus, for eight years when a debilitating flare spurred me to research better ways of managing my condition. I was tired of feeling powerless and not knowing how I was going to feel from one day to the next. My research led me to the Paleo diet, the starting point from which I uncovered a wealth of scientific research explaining how certain foods can be highly inflammatory and have the potential to set off a whole cascade of autoimmune reactions while other foods are a powerful ally in healing an overreactive immune system. I used my expertise as a medical researcher to compile scientific evidence with the goal of maximizing the therapeutic potential of diet and founded the Autoimmune Protocol (AIP).

As I began to heal, I decided to create an outlet where I could share my research. In 2011, my blog ThePaleoMom.com was born. Never did I imagine that the Autoimmune Protocol would develop into what it has become today. I'm proud and delighted to see it gain traction as a recognized means to remove stress and inflammation, regulate the immune system, balance hormones, reverse chronic symptoms, and heal the gut.

What also gives me immense pride is the number of bloggers and health practitioners who not only support my work but are helping thousands of people fight their own autoimmune battles by creating resources and sharing their own personal stories. One such advocate is Kate Jay, who has been an asset to this community since 2014, both for her creative, nutrient-rich recipes and her work as a Functional Nutritional Therapy Practitioner and AIP Certified Coach.

Such is the strength of this movement that you will find several books offering recipes compliant with the elimination phase of the Autoimmune Protocol. However, *The Autoimmune Protocol Reintroduction Cookbook* is the first book devoted to the second phase—the reintroduction process. This book has been needed for some time now, and I know it will be appreciated by so many. I'm thrilled that Kate brought it to the community.

The essential self-discovery process of reintroductions is key to identifying personal autoimmune triggers, dietary expansion, and homing in on an individualized optimal diet for lifelong health. Yet, the subject of reintroductions is one that many approach with a degree of anxiety or that they may be unwilling to approach it at all. Having been through the protocol herself, Kate understands the overwhelm that can happen, and she uses her nutritional and AIP coaching experience to gently guide the reader along the journey. She prepares the reader by reinforcing continued intake of nutrient-dense foods. She then offers suggestions for achieving improved digestive health, as well as developing a mindset of success rather than failure. She gives sound advice on when and how to approach each of the reintroduction stages for the best possible chance of success. Preparation is key, and Kate ensures that the reader is well equipped and encouraged to move forward when the time is right. Her friendly, enthusiastic approach will ensure the reader feels understood and supported, even congratulated throughout the journey.

The microorganisms in our guts help to maintain the delicate balance required by our immune systems, keeping the various populations of immune cells in check and modulating their activity. In fact, gut dysbiosis (an unhealthy gut microbiome) is present in every autoimmune disease in which its presence has been investigated. Maintaining a healthy balance in the immune system is therefore reliant on having a healthy gut microbiome. My most recent research has found that some non-Paleo foods—such as oats, split peas, lentils, chickpeas, and rice—are of huge benefit to the gut microbiome and can certainly be included as an adjunct to a Paleo diet. I have added these foods into my own diet and encourage my readers to do the same, following the recommended reintroduction procedure, of course. You'll find some delicious recipes using these ingredients in the later chapters of this book.

It's wonderful to see that nearly all the recipes in this guide can be modified to suit those who are coconut-free, need to incorporate low FODMAPs, or have yet to leave the elimination phase. This book will appeal to you and your friends and family, whether on an "elimination diet" or not. In fact, don't even mention it because they won't know the difference anyway—the recipes are that good!

A large part of succeeding on the Autoimmune Protocol is the ability to find joy in life, and that includes taking into account the foods we eat. It can be hard to make simple yet delicious food when we are dealing with health challenges. But believe me, you are going to love the recipes in this book. With Kate's stunning photography, each one is a feast for the eyes as well as the taste buds. If you find joy from the comfort of treats, prepare to indulge in the most delicious cakes, cookies, and desserts, all created to optimize nutrients without causing blood sugar spikes and ruining your hard work.

In short, Kate is a talented chef whose book is the gift the autoimmune community has been waiting for. You are in good hands, so prepare to be reunited with your favorite foods in a safe, well thought out, highly flavorful and healing way.

—Dr. Sarah Ballantyne, Ph.D.

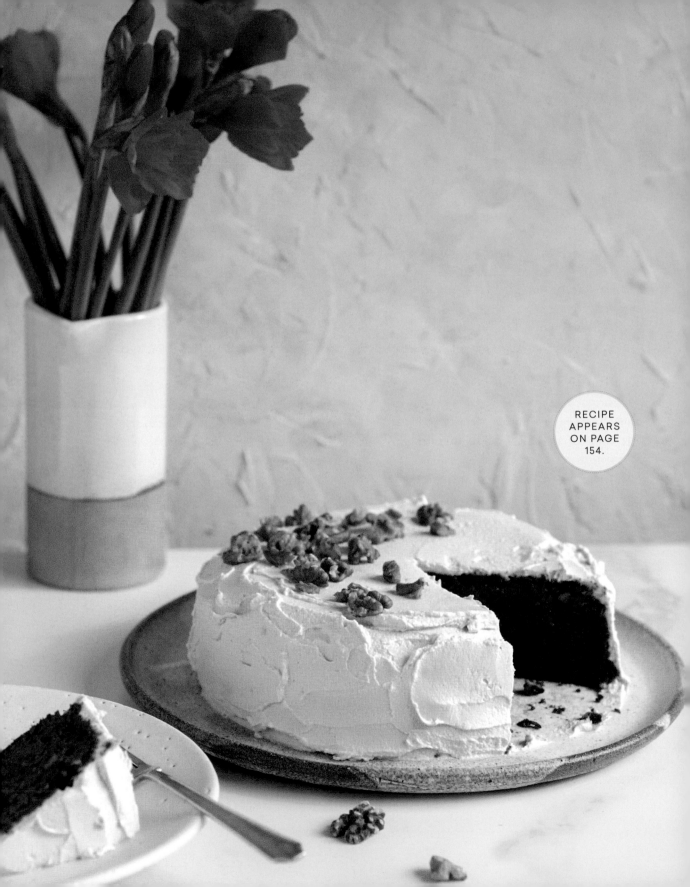

RECIPE
APPEARS
ON PAGE
154.

INTRODUCTION

WHEN I WAS SMALL, my grandparents came to live with us. My grandmother was severely disabled with an autoimmune disease called rheumatoid arthritis, which manifests in the joints. She couldn't do a single thing for herself, so all her needs were taken care of by my grandfather and my parents. In constant pain, she was housebound and miserable. Several decades later I clearly remember her calling out to the Lord to take her.

My brother was diagnosed with terminal cancer in 2008 and given five weeks to live. Those weeks were by far the worst of my life. Seeing a fit, strong man reduced to a helpless shell within weeks and being told there was nothing we could do—it was devastating. As predicted, five weeks later he died. Cancer is the cruelest of diseases; the wreckage left behind was enormous. There's no doubt that chronic stress takes a destructive toll. Within a year my mother had a heart attack resulting in bypass surgery. Looking back, I now recognize my father showing very early signs of the Alzheimer's disease that he has fully succumbed to.

I developed signs and symptoms of dysfunction before I'd even left the hospice that final time. I'd already been living with hypothyroidism since 1997; now joint pain, crippling anxiety, depression, panic attacks, and frequent occurrences of irritable bowel syndrome (IBS) became a way of life for me for the next six years. In 2014 I noticed symmetrical swelling in my thumb and wrist joints, and pain in my hips, ankles, and feet. My joints were stiff, red, and warm to the touch, and, sure enough, I had elevated markers for rheumatoid arthritis.

Despite being waved away by my doctor with the words "Keep calm and carry on" and "Keep the British stiff upper lip," I decided to advocate for my own health. I spent hours on the computer until I came across the Autoimmune Protocol. There were only a small handful of AIP bloggers back in 2014, but I found posts from people who had achieved astonishing success, and I knew I wanted to be part of it. I found Mickey Trescott's *Autoimmune Paleo* blog (now *Autoimmune Wellness*) at a time when she was about to release her first cookbook. The timing couldn't have been better.

So, I changed my diet and lifestyle, and within days my morning stiffness and joint pain disappeared. Not long afterward my brain fog lifted, and within a few months my swelling was gone, along with my autoimmune marker.

My brother left his savings to me, and eight years after his death I enrolled with the Nutritional Therapy Association, knowing that was where his money belonged. If I couldn't help him, his legacy was going to enable me to help others instead. After graduation I went straight into the first AIP Certified Coach Training Program led by Dr. Sarah Ballantyne, Mickey

Trescott, and Angie Alt. From there I completed yet more courses to satiate my passion for learning about health and wellness.

Autoimmune diseases occur when the immune system mistakenly targets our own healthy cells and tissues. The AIP is a diet that temporarily excludes foods known to increase inflammation and overstimulate the immune system, while also adding nutrient-rich foods and reducing empty calories. It's about using food and lifestyle as medicine.

AIP is not a cure; rather, it gives the body an opportunity to reset the immune system. You then slowly reintroduce foods into your diet while carefully watching for reactions. The body wants to heal. It just needs the tools to do so. Taking away the stressors and bolstering the defenses helps to equip the body to do its job.

Note that the reintroduction information is the equivalent of a starter course for you. Use this book as a template and be sure to reach out to a practitioner skilled in the AIP if you feel troubleshooting is necessary. Don't let your diet become more restricted due to the emergence of new food sensitivities. This is a sign your immune system is still on high alert and you need to look for root issues while navigating the process on a more bio-individual level. Don't forget that autoimmune disease is a diagnosis, not a cause.

I started my AIP blog, *Healing Family Eats,* because I love food and needed motivation to stick with the elimination phase. Increasingly, though, a common reason for my clients reaching out to me is AIP reintroductions: Either they are timid about starting, or they have tried and, in their words, "failed." I prefer to see it as a message that your body isn't quite ready and after some fine-tuning, it's a different story.

While there are plenty of recipe resources available for the elimination phase of the protocol, finding recipes to help with reintroductions is more challenging. In this book I share recipes developed with reintroductions in mind. The majority are also easily adaptable for those still on the elimination phase.

Changing your diet does not mean giving up on flavor. When you put aside the foods that are causing you to inflame and instead give your body the nutrients it craves, eating gets a whole lot better—as does your health. Above all, enjoy. Happy cooking, and happy healing!

HOW TO USE
THIS BOOK

WHETHER YOU HAVE several reintroductions under your belt or have yet to start the process, it couldn't be better timing that you have found this book! My aim is to encourage and support you as you navigate the reintroduction phase of the AIP. The recipes have been developed with gentle reintroductions in mind, taking you through all four stages, with the ultimate goal of you finding your own unique template.

You should do this when you feel truly ready. Just keep in mind that it's important not to get stuck by fear of undoing all your hard work and resist initiating the reintroduction process at all. If you're not quite ready for reintroductions, simply follow the modifications and slip in the relevant reintroduction food when the time is right. The majority of recipes are easily adapted to be elimination phase compliant.

Here are some things to remember as you use this book:

- Always read the recipe through from beginning to end before getting started.

- Read through the Kitchen Basics section on page 10. There's a lot of information related to getting the most out of the recipes in this book, such as useful tips and how-tos.

- Some recipes suggest soaking, dehydrating, and even sprouting ingredients beforehand. You don't have to do this, but it is strongly recommended. The aim is to make the reintroduction foods easier on your digestive system, and therefore more likely to bring you success.

- Batch cooking recipes where possible will make your life easier and minimize time spent in the kitchen.

Short for Fermentable Oligosaccharides, Disaccharides, Monosaccharides, and Polyols, FODMAP refers to groups of carbohydrates and sugar alcohols that are not completely absorbed in the gut but are fermented by bacteria living there. This fermentation causes a range of digestive symptoms, including gas, bloating, and abdominal pain.

AIP COMPLIANT Recipes can be made elimination phase compliant by following the tips.

FREEZER-FRIENDLY Some or all parts can be frozen. These are marked.

LOW FODMAP Either the entire recipe is low FODMAP or it can be adapted using the information provided.

COCONUT-FREE Recipes are automatically coconut-free or can be adapted using the information provided.

KITCHEN BASICS

WHEN READING THE RECIPES in this book, keep in mind the following guidelines:

- All eggs are large size and organic.

- Lemon juice should be freshly squeezed when possible to extract maximum nutrients and flavor.

- Coconut milk is always full-fat and additive-free. I like Aroy-D brand. Always check the ingredients of any brand you choose; they can change over time.

- Good quality extra virgin olive oil, coconut oil, and avocado oil are the most stable plant oils for higher temperature cooking. Rotate cooking oils with animal fats from grass-fed, pasture-raised animals. Avoid processed seed oils as these are highly inflammatory.

- Check vanilla extract to be sure it is soy-free and certified gluten-free. If you are on the elimination phase you will want to buy alcohol-free. Alternatively substitute ½ teaspoon ground powder for each teaspoon of extract.

- A word about palm shortening: I have seen too many videos of the devastation caused by deforestation due to logging and palm oil plantations. I fear that what has happened in Southeast Asia may repeat itself in Africa and Latin America. So, while Greenpeace and the Roundtable on Sustainable Palm Oil (RSPO) are in disagreement over its sustainability, I don't use palm shortening in my recipes. I suggest lard as a good substitute in baking; coconut oil often works well too, particularly in cakes. If you don't agree with me, palm shortening can be used interchangeably with the aforementioned lard in baking recipes.

BASIC RECIPES AND HOW-TOS

bone broth
(makes 3 to 4 quarts [3 to 4 liters])

1. Place 2 to 3 pounds (about 1 to 1.25 kg) of meat bones or poultry carcasses in a stockpot. Add a splash of apple cider vinegar to draw out the minerals. (Note: Meat bones can be used several times until they start to crumble. Use poultry bones only once.)

2. Add 4 to 5 chicken feet to poultry carcasses to achieve a more gelatinous broth for extra gut healing.

3. Cover with filtered water and bring to a boil. Reduce the temperature and simmer gently for 12 to 24 hours, the longer the better. Alternatively, you can use a pressure cooker. Cook on manual for 2 hours with a slow release.

4. Cool and portion the broth into containers and refrigerate or freeze until needed.

gelatin egg (makes 2)

1. Put 2 tablespoons (20 g) of grass-fed gelatin in a small bowl. Put 1 teaspoon apple cider vinegar, and 3 tablespoons (45 ml) hot water in a separate small bowl.

2. Pour the liquid onto the gelatin and whisk until frothy.

3. Use the gelatin egg as instructed in the recipe.

coconut cream

1. Put a can of coconut milk in the refrigerator the night before you want to use it. The coconut cream will rise to the top.

2. Turn the can upside down and open it with a can opener.

3. Pour off the water and reserve it for use in smoothies or sauces. The remainder of the can is coconut cream.

three ways to separate an egg

-   Hard-boil the egg and separate the yolk from the white, discarding the film surrounding the yolk.

-   Crack a raw egg into your cupped fingers or a slotted spoon. Very gently run cold water over the yolk to wash off the white.

-   Over a small bowl, crack open an egg so you are holding half a shell in each hand. Transfer the yolk back and forth, allowing the white to fall into the bowl. This method is only recommended if you tolerate both the yolk and white.

NOTE **Surplus yolks and whites can be put separately into ice cube trays and frozen. If you freeze them individually and store them in containers or bags, you will always know how many you have.**

prepare rice to reduce arsenic

1. Thoroughly rinse the rice in a bowl or sieve until water runs clear.

2. Soak the rice for at least 8 hours in a bowl of filtered water with a splash of apple cider vinegar.

3. Drain the rice and rinse again. Put it in a pan with plenty of filtered water and cook until ready. Transfer the rice to a sieve.

4. Boil a kettle full of water and pour it over the rice to drain off residual toxins.

NOTE **The rice cooks much more quickly using this method.**

SOAKING AND SPROUTING

Soaking nuts, seeds, and legumes makes them easier on the digestive system, and their nutrients more bioavailable. This is important because many of these foods have antinutrients (e.g., lectins, phytates, and saponins) in them. These block mineral uptake and cause intestinal permeability. Sprouting your own is much more cost effective, but you can purchase sprouted nuts, seeds, and legumes and their flours online.

Soak nuts and seeds overnight in filtered water with a large pinch of sea salt to neutralize enzyme inhibitors. Cashews and macadamia nuts need to soak for a maximum of six hours or they go slimy. After soaking, rinse them well and then place in a sprouting jar or tray. Then rinse twice daily until sprouted.

Seeds take only one to four days to sprout but not all nuts can be sprouted. Skinless raw almonds are an exception.

	SOAK	ADD TO WATER	SPROUT	DEHYDRATE
almonds	overnight	sea salt	3 days if raw	12–24 hours
cashews	4–6 hours		N/A	12–24 hours
hazelnuts	overnight	sea salt	N/A	12–24 hours
macadamia	6 hours	sea salt	N/A	12–24 hours
pecans	overnight	sea salt	N/A	12–24 hours
pistachios	4–6 hours	sea salt	N/A	12–24 hours
walnuts	overnight	sea salt	N/A	12–24 hours
hemp seeds	N/A		N/A	N/A
pumpkin seeds	overnight	sea salt	12–18 hours	12–24 hours
sesame seeds	overnight	sea salt	2–3 days	12–24 hours
sunflower seeds	overnight	sea salt	12–18 hours	12–24 hours

A dehydrator is useful when introducing nuts and seeds. To dehydrate them, pat dry with paper towels and set a dehydrator to 105°F (41°C) for twelve to twenty-four hours until they are completely dry and crisp. If you don't have a dehydrator, place them in a single layer on parchment-lined baking trays and oven-dry at 150°F (66°C) or lower, stirring occasionally for at least twelve hours. Be aware that oven-drying destroys valuable enzymes, but it will rid enzyme inhibitors.

Store in the refrigerator. Even if you intend to roast or toast the nuts and seeds it is good practice to dehydrate them first. Thoroughly drying them out prevents mold from building up inside.

Soaking legumes in three times the amount of filtered water before cooking will greatly improve their digestibility. Presoaked lentils can be successfully sprouted in three days and then refrigerated in a lidded container.

Pressure cooking considerably decreases the lectin content in soaked legumes and only takes ten to fifteen minutes at high pressure, depending on the type.

To cook the soaked legumes on the stove top, add twice the amount of water and bring to a simmer. Cook for one and a half to two hours.

Legumes roughly double their bulk once soaked and cooked (3/4 cup of dried legumes = 15-ounce can, drained).

Adding a strip of kombu seaweed adds minerals and further improves digestion. Eden Foods is one of the few manufacturers that presoak and pressure cook their legumes with kombu, so you will find these easier to digest than those brands that do not. The canning process denatures nutrients and is less cost effective than preparing your own. Note that legumes are lower in FODMAPs when canned.

For more information on soaking and sprouting, visit the Weston A. Price Foundation at www.westonaprice.org.

GRAINS AND LEGUMES

	SOAK	ADD TO WATER	SPROUT	DEHYDRATE
oats	24 hours	apple cider vinegar/ lemon juice	N/A	N/A
rice	overnight	apple cider vinegar/ lemon juice	N/A	N/A
wild rice	overnight	apple cider vinegar/ lemon juice	N/A	N/A
cannellini beans	24 hours	N/A	2–3 days	N/A
chickpeas/ garbanzo beans	24 hours	lemon juice	2–3 days	N/A
great northern beans	24 hours	lemon juice	2–3 days	N/A
lentils	8–10 hours	apple cider vinegar/ lemon juice	2–3 days	N/A
peanuts	overnight	sea salt	N/A	12–24 hours
split peas	10 hours	pinch baking soda	2–3 days	N/A

USEFUL CONVERSIONS

weight

½ oz = 15 g
1 oz = 30 g
2 oz = 55 g
3 oz = 85 g
4 oz = ¼ lb = 110 g
5 oz = 140 g
6 oz = 170 g
7 oz = 200 g
8 oz = ½ lb = 225 g
12 oz = ¾ lb = 340 g
13 oz = 370 g
14 oz = 400 g
15 oz = 425 g
1 lb = 450 g
1¼ lb = 560 g
1½ lb = 675 g
2 lb = 900 g

length

¼ inch = 6 mm
½ inch = 1 cm
¾ inch = 2 cm
1 inch = 2.5 cm
8 inches = 20 cm
9 inches = 23 cm

liquid measurements

1 teaspoon = 5 ml
1 tablespoon = 15 ml or 3 teaspoons
¼ cup = 60 ml
⅓ cup = 80 ml
½ cup = 125 ml
1 cup = 250 ml
¼ pint = 150 ml = 5 fl oz
½ pint = 290 ml = 10 fl oz
1 pint = 570 ml = 20 fl oz

oven temperatures

275°F (140°C, or gas mark 1)
300°F (150°C, or gas mark 2)
325°F (170°C, or gas mark 3)
350°F (175°C, or gas mark 4)
375°F (190°C, or gas mark 5)
400°F (200°C, or gas mark 6)
425°F (220°C, or gas mark 7)
450°F (230°C, or gas mark 8)
475°F (240°C, or gas mark 9)
500°F (260°C, or gas mark 10)

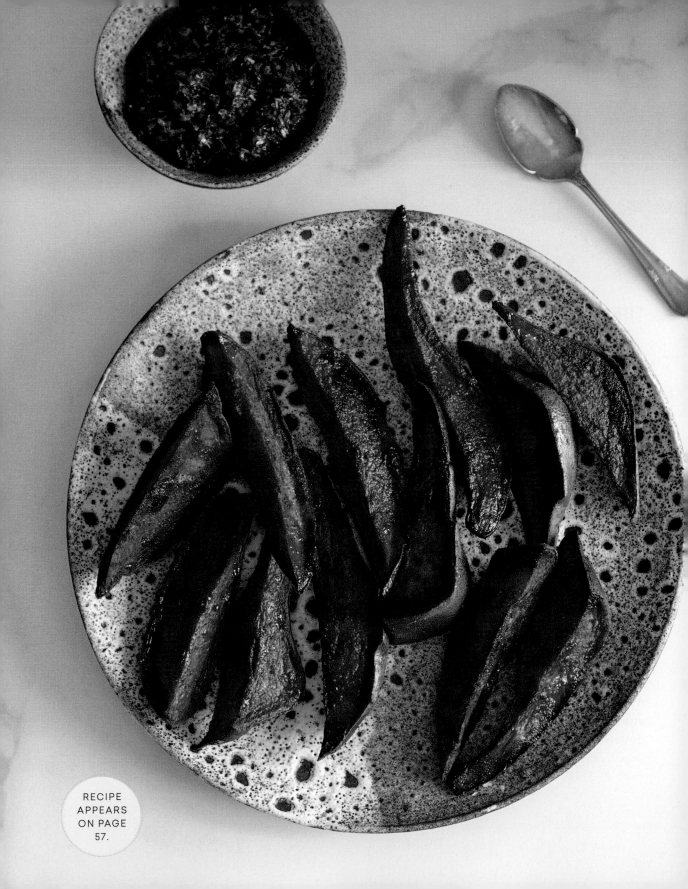

RECIPE
APPEARS
ON PAGE
57.

CHAPTER ONE

THE
AUTOIMMUNE PROTOCOL (AIP)

OUR IMMUNE SYSTEM is supposed to work 24/7 to protect us from foreign invaders such as bacteria, viruses, parasites, and other pathogens. Autoimmune diseases occur when our immune system mistakenly turns and targets our own healthy cells and tissues instead. This happens as a result of the immune system releasing proteins called autoantibodies.

Constant assaults by these autoantibodies leave the body incapable of defense. And, if the attack doesn't stop and the body isn't adequately equipped for the fight, inflammation increases and cellular destruction occurs. To quote Dr. Sarah Ballantyne, in her essential book *The Paleo Approach*, "all autoimmune diseases are caused by a betrayal of the immune system."

Research shows that genetics plays only a small part in our chances of having an autoimmune disease. Most of the risk comes from environmental triggers, diet, and lifestyle.

WHAT IS THE AIP?

The AIP is a temporary elimination diet that excludes foods known to increase inflammation and overstimulate the immune system. It also focuses on putting nutrients back in, and addresses lifestyle components to reduce and reverse symptoms, heal the gut, and rebalance hormones. After a significant amount of healing, foods are slowly and methodically reintroduced while watching for reactions.

The AIP is a healing diet based on the Paleo template aimed at people living with autoimmune disease or undiagnosed chronic inflammatory symptoms. Loren Cordain, Ph.D., author of *The Paleo Diet,* and Robb Wolf, author of *The Paleo Solution,* originally set the AIP wheels in motion as a primal healing diet. However, it was Dr. Sarah Ballantyne, herself diagnosed with several autoimmune diseases, who made the AIP into the groundbreaking protocol it is today.

The AIP focuses on driving down inflammation in the body and reducing symptoms, using food and lifestyle as medicine. This means removing stressors that come from inflammatory foods, and addressing poor stress management, lack of sleep, and under- or over-exercising.

Of equal importance is what we put into our body. When we have chronic symptoms of disease, we are malnourished and it is essential to prioritize nutrient-rich foods and minimize empty calories, such as sugar-laden treats. This combination helps heal the damage to our gut and encourage our bodies to strive for wellness. Once this happens, we can start the process of reintroducing eliminated foods with the goal to achieve the least restrictive way of eating possible.

AIP has evolved since its inception, in line with Dr. Ballantyne's continued research. For instance, in 2019 foods such as coffee, chocolate, high-protein dairy, chia seeds, cashews, lentils, and chickpeas, to name but a few, were moved to earlier reintroduction stages due to their ability to increase beneficial bacteria at the expense of opportunistic strains, or their positive effect on the gut microbiome.

The results of this research encouraged me to attempt several reintroductions of my own while writing this book. Most were successful, and even those that did not go as well gave me a better understanding of what my body can handle. Knowledge is key, and it is a rewarding exercise to listen to our body's needs and accept that some things take time. As long as we maintain a focus on nutrition, the chances of later success are increased.

THE AIP IS NOT A "CURE"

There are more than one hundred recognized autoimmune diseases and a further forty are suspected to be related. Statistics show that once you have one autoimmune disease, the risk of having more increases. There is no cure for autoimmune disease. Doctors will prescribe medication to help treat or manage it. While we are fortunate to have medications to deal with pain and symptom management (and there's nothing wrong with taking them), they do come with potential health risks of their own.

WHY DO THE AIP?

We are all extremely lucky to have allopathic medicine at our fingertips, and there's no doubt it has a crucial role to play. But it is important to keep in mind that food, together with lifestyle factors, is truly the greatest medicine of all. Indeed, it was Hippocrates, the Greek physician known as the "Father of Medicine" and whose oath is still sworn by all new physicians, who said "Let food be thy medicine and medicine be thy food."

Dr. Tom O'Bryan, author of *The Autoimmune Fix,* says, "Every forkful of what you put in your mouth is either inflammatory or anti-inflammatory. Make wise choices." When it comes to autoimmune disease, a wise choice can make the difference between how symptomatic you are and whether you calm your immune system or cause it to flare. With nutrition and lifestyle in mind, thousands of people with autoimmune disease have used the AIP to achieve positive, life-changing results. Scientific studies, fronted by Mickey Trescott and Angie Alt of Autoimmune Wellness, now back the AIP as a credible modality for healing (see Resources, page 202). To date, positive studies on the efficacy of the AIP have been conducted on patients with inflammatory bowel disease (IBD) and Hashimoto's thyroiditis. Current studies on eczema and psoriasis are being conducted to confirm the benefits of the AIP in supporting these conditions.

IT'S NOT YOUR FAULT!

Dr. Francis Collins, an American physician-geneticist who discovered the genes associated with a number of diseases, said, "Genetics loads the gun; environment pulls the trigger." Simply put, if your family has a history of diabetes, cancer, autoimmune disease, yes, you are probably more predisposed to follow suit. But you are in control of your gene expression: Genes can be switched on; they can also be switched off.

Most of your risk comes from your environment and lifestyle. Modern-day stressors come from financial or family pressures, rushing to get the children to school, caring for elderly parents, sitting in daily traffic, or perhaps preparing for work meetings or business trips. All while running a home.

Our downtime comes with stressors, too. We take in more toxins on a daily basis than we are

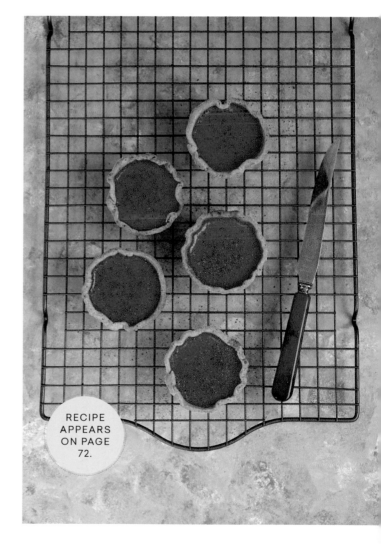

RECIPE APPEARS ON PAGE 72.

able to eliminate, which overburdens our detoxification pathways. Our days revolve around technology that comes with health warnings. Blue light from screens and indoor light bulbs confuse our brains' inner clocks, which then disrupt our circadian rhythms, resulting in sleep issues.

Our stressors also come from what we eat. Chemical pesticides, GMOs, and other modern farming methods have changed food production dramatically. Conventionally raised livestock is subjected to multiple rounds of hormones and antibiotics, which are routinely served on our dinner plates along with the meat and vegetables.

THE IMPORTANCE OF GOOD DIGESTION

The body needs to go through many processes to break down, absorb, and use the nutrients in our food. This starts with digestion, which is the foundational piece of our health and wellness jigsaw puzzle. But to digest our food, it is essential that we are in a parasympathetic state of "rest and digest." Our ancestors prayed and gave thanks while sitting in front of their plates: Showing gratitude encouraged them to slow down and prepare for digestion.

Today, we live in a world where everything is done quickly and cheaply. We even eat our food quickly. Many of us eat while multitasking—perhaps working at the office desk, in front of our screens, watching television, or driving in the car. Even our children are often given just a few short minutes to eat their lunch at school.

Our bodies are amazing, and they make priorities, just as our minds do. When you are stressed and rushed, your body pools its resources at the expense of digestion, detoxification, reproduction, and, yes, immune function. All this uses up a lot of energy, and it depletes the nutrients needed to keep us in balance. When we live with constant stress, we absorb fewer nutrients and become yet more depleted, so we ultimately fall into degeneration, dysfunction, and disease.

Underlying infections from pathogens, emotional stress, and exposure to chemicals and other toxins result in nutrient depletion and food sensitivities, which are highly destructive to our guts. The gut wall is only the thickness of an eyelid and soon becomes permeable enough to allow food particles and toxins to push their way through to the blood stream, which activates the immune system still further. Over time, the immune system may target foods that have the potential to switch from being medicine to the body's poison.

LET FOOD BE THY "PRIMARY" MEDICINE

"You are what you eat" is actually a half-truth. More accurately, it is "you are what you eat, digest, and absorb"! The reality is that the most pristine diet in the world won't help much if you can't digest it, so allow me to set you on the right path.

I love a good analogy, and this is the one I give my clients: Do you remember those marble runs that you likely played with as a child, or maybe watch your children or grandchildren enjoying today? They're a lot of fun, when you place the marble on the top layer and watch it speed along toward a hole in the run that sends it down onto the next level, and so on. Without that hole, the marble won't go anywhere because it needs a trigger to help it along the process. Now let's talk about digestion.

Many people think that digestion begins in the stomach or the mouth, but it actually starts in the brain. The sight, smell, sound, and anticipation of food starts the process before you've put anything in your mouth. When the brain is engaged into expecting food, it signals the release of saliva. As you chew thoroughly, enzymes in the saliva break down the nutrients and digest a mind-blowing 30 percent of carbohydrates while they're still in your mouth. As this triggers the release of acid from the stomach walls, the digestion of protein occurs. The same acid disinfects the stomach and kills pathogens before they can set up camp. Meanwhile, the gallbladder secretes bile to help break down fats and remove toxins through the gastrointestinal (GI) tract. The contents of the stomach pass through to the small intestine where they are bathed in enzymes and bicarbonates that neutralize the acidity and prevent the small intestine from burning. All this time nutrients are being absorbed through the gut, including a final attempt in the colon before the elimination of waste. So, with the marble run analogy in mind, if you don't insert the correct pieces of the track right from the start, you've got a challenge on your hands to finish the game.

REST AND DIGEST

Because digestion uses up a lot of energy, we need to make it as easy as possible on our digestive system. Try this simple, unobtrusive breathing exercise to relax you. I also like to do this if I feel anxious; it works like a charm.

1. Start with a deep breath in through the nose and out through the mouth.

2. Using a finger on your right hand, push it gently against your right nostril to plug it up.

3. With mouth closed, slowly breathe in through the left nostril.

4. Mouth still closed, slowly breathe out through the left nostril.

5. Repeat four or five times, or until you feel yourself switch to a relaxed state.

Start with a few deep breaths before eating to switch into a "rest and digest" state. Ideally chew each mouthful of food thirty times to break it down and allow saliva to do its job. If that sounds like a tall order, start with ten chews and build up over time. Put your fork down between bites to encourage you to slow down. Be aware of saliva wrapping around and mixing in with your food, and only swallow when the contents of your mouth feel like soup. Remember, the less work your body has to do, the more energy it supplies for regeneration, repair, and all the fun things in life.

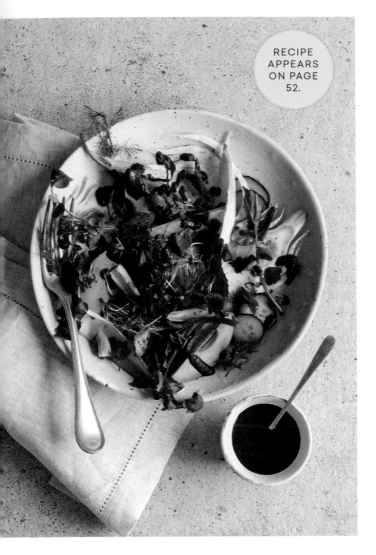

RECIPE APPEARS ON PAGE 52.

- Choose grass-fed and pasture-raised meats and wild-caught fish. All contain more omega-3 fatty acids than when conventionally reared and are far less likely to create inflammation.

- Organ meat is strongly encouraged because it is so nutrient rich. Liver is particularly valuable on a healing diet because that's where nutrients are stored. Note that predatory animals will invariably start with the organ meats before heading on to the muscle.

- If you really can't tolerate the idea of organ meats, you may be pleased to know that shellfish is classed as organ meat, because you eat the whole thing. This is equally true of crickets, which are crustaceans (avoid if you have a shellfish allergy). In small amounts, they are delicious in baked goods.

- Organic vegetables are grown without chemical pesticides and fertilizers, and therefore are much healthier options. Vegetables, predominantly non-starchy varieties, should make up the bulk of your meal. Dr. Sarah Ballantyne recommends a minimum of 8 cups of veggies a day (measured raw). Always remember to "eat the rainbow": Fill your plate with a mix of fiber-rich leafy greens and salad vegetables, and cruciferous, sulfur-rich vegetables. Roots and tubers provide our starchy carbohydrates.

- Fruits are packed with nutrients and fiber, and many are rich in antioxidants. Keep daily intake below 40 grams of fructose, which is roughly three to five servings depending on the fruit. Again, choose organic when possible.

CHOOSE NUTRIENT-DENSE FOOD

Nutrient density matters. Many vitamin-, mineral-, and enzyme-rich foods are eliminated on the AIP, so it is crucial to concentrate on nutrient density. We need these nutrients to help heal the gut lining.

- Broccoli sprouts and other microgreens are nutritional powerhouses, more so than the fully grown plants. They take just a matter of days to grow at home.

- Treat herbs as vegetables and add large amounts to salads or right at the end of cooking.

- Put sea vegetables on your list, too. They are a rich source of minerals that are hard to get from our over-cultivated soils. I love dulse and kelp flakes sprinkled over soups and sautéed veggies, and I also often incorporate them into my liver paté.

- Dr. Sarah Ballantyne recently elevated mushrooms to superfood status, qualifying as their own essential food group due to their highly beneficial effect on the microbiome.

- Fermented foods, such as sauerkraut, kimchi, and beet kvass, all feed the beneficial bacteria residing in our gut, which In turn make nutrients for us. Recipes for these can be found in this book (pages 77, 123, and 201).

- Bone broth (see Kitchen Basics, page 10) contains valuable concentrations of amino acids, including glycine and proline, which promote digestion, detoxification, and overall healing.

Fats should be sourced from grass-fed, pasture-raised animals, fatty-rich fish, and plant oils such as avocado, coconut, and, most importantly, olive oil. Fat plays important roles in the body, such as aiding the absorption of fat-soluble vitamins, blood sugar regulation, and balancing hormones. Good-quality animal fats are essential, because toxins are stored in fat cells.

Buying the best-quality food will yield the most intense nutrients, but, sadly, this tends to be more expensive. Check out the "Clean Fifteen" and "Dirty Dozen" lists from the Environmental Working Group (see Resources, page 202) to find out the conventionally grown fruits and vegetables that are safest to buy and the twelve that should be organic. But truly, don't let cost be a deal breaker in doing the AIP. Do the best your budget will allow. You are going to reap rewards no matter what.

A word about desserts and treats: Although hardly nutrient dense, they should not be seen as the enemy. Goodness knows, there's enough guilt surrounding food as it is, and part of the healing process involves finding contentment. The selection you'll find in this book is deliberately low in sweeteners and should be seen as something to enjoy on an occasional basis, rather than a daily occurrence.

THE AIP IS A LIFESTYLE PROTOCOL

Nutrient-dense foods play a powerful role in healing the gut, but we need to take lifestyle factors into account, too. Optimizing sleep and stress management, incorporating adequate movement that doesn't tax the gut, and focusing on the mind–body connection, are all necessary for the healing process.

Improve your sleep: Detoxification, repair, and regeneration all occur when we sleep. While we were designed to deal with some stress, chronic long-term stress increases intestinal permeability (also known as leaky gut) that impacts our whole-body system. Remember that time spent

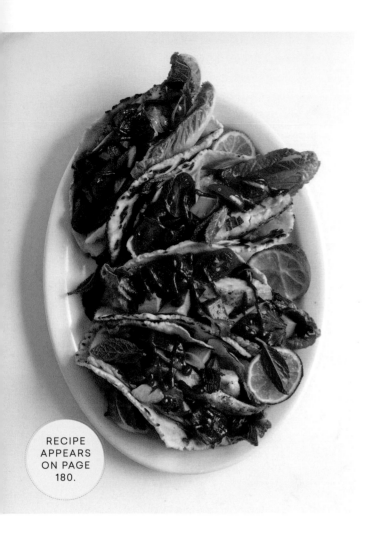

RECIPE
APPEARS
ON PAGE
180.

have known sensitivities to them. Be cautious of manufacturers who claim their products are "all natural." Remember mercury, lead, and aluminum are naturally occurring minerals!

Manage stress: Recognizing what it takes to keep you calm and grounded is an important part of healing. As is honoring your emotions by connecting with people who make you feel loved and supported, and minimizing (even cutting off) time spent with those you find physically and emotionally draining. Learning to trust in your body's ability to regenerate and repair goes a long way toward healing your mind, body, and soul.

Find emotional support: After receiving a diagnosis, many people go through a lengthened grieving process, or they push it out of mind and deny its existence. Some may have the added challenge of family, friends, or work colleagues not fully understanding their daily struggles, because autoimmune disease is an invisible illness. Like you, perhaps, I've been told to suck it up and move on. That concept never resonated with me. Instead I took comfort in seeing my future as following a different, albeit unplanned, path. It's important to deal with these emotions and challenges so that you can fully embrace healing. Take time to grieve and then reach acceptance, seeking professional help if you feel that's unobtainable. It is then that you will truly step up the healing process.

TRANSITIONING TO THE AIP

There are two ways to approach transitioning to the AIP: Some like to dive in; others need time to ease into it. Either can work well, and you should

under stress forces our body to think we're under attack and calls on our adrenal glands to help out when necessary. All these factors determine the health of our immune system.

Reduce your toxic load: Help your health by removing toxic exposure from household cleaning fluids, personal care, and hygiene products. Our skin is our largest organ—check that personal products are also gluten-free. Rule out ingredients such as soy, dairy, and corn if you

choose the path that works best for you. If you are highly motivated, super organized, good at holding yourself accountable, and have a lot of support, you may feel that cold turkey is the approach for you. Be aware that an immediate change may result in an increase in symptoms as your body adjusts. It might even put you into a flare.

Adopting a slower approach over several weeks will take longer to reach the full elimination phase. But it may be the best choice if you don't have the flexibility or planning skills to make it happen quickly. Easing into this phase will also be better if giving up your favorite foods is very challenging. A slow elimination, in which you replace foods to be avoided with those that fuel healing, may help you recognize which foods you are sensitive to. If this is the case, it's actually very useful information, and you'll also know to leave those until much later in the reintroduction process.

What works for one person isn't necessarily right for the next. Remember, the important thing is that you get there in the end. Whichever transition style suits you, print out the lists of foods to avoid and include. Reduce their size, laminate, and keep them with you. Or have the information stored as your cell phone screen saver so you always have it at hand.

Setting aside three to four hours once a week to cook a few recipes for the freezer will build up a welcome supply of ready meals for those days when you can't or don't want to cook. If you prefer, three or four times a week cook double or triple the amount you're making for dinner. If you portion out and freeze the leftovers, you'll have a good stash in no time.

Get involved with the AIP online community for support and connection with people who truly understand what you're going through. There are a lot of us out there.

Above all, remember the importance of self-care to reduce feeling overwhelmed. Remind yourself you can do anything for thirty days, and it takes just twenty-one of them to form a new habit. If you need to lengthen your time on the elimination phase, you've already got your routine sorted. There is never a perfect time to start or get back on track, and imperfect action is always better than none at all.

AIP IS NOT A FOREVER DIET

The AIP is intended to be a temporary diet to allow your body to heal and to discern which foods provoke immune reactions. Being faithful to the elimination phase for a minimum of thirty days will help calm immune function, as well as reduce inflammation and other symptoms. It will also start to heal the gut lining and repair the damage done as a result of your mistaken immune system.

The reality, though, is that it's hard to say exactly how long it will take. If you think about the length of time it has taken from those first symptoms to receiving your diagnosis, it's unrealistic to expect an overnight fix. You'd be wise to count on the elimination phase lasting up to ninety days, and possibly more. If after ninety days you don't see the improvement you were hoping for, consider reaching out to a skilled practitioner who can help you dig deeper toward the root cause.

FOODS TO EAT

It's important to eat enough food. The AIP isn't low-carb but rather than eating starchy carbohydrates from bread, pizza, and pasta, these now come from increasing your vegetable intake with sweet potatoes, parsnips, plantains, and winter squashes and the like as your new filler foods.

meat	beef, bison, chicken, duck, elk, goat, lamb, pork, rabbit, turkey, venison
organ meat	bone broth, gizzard, heart, kidney, liver, tongue
seafood	anchovy, arctic char, bass, cod, haddock, halibut, herring, mackerel, monkfish, salmon, sardine, snapper, sole, swordfish, tilapia, trout, tuna
shellfish	clam, crab, lobster, mussels, octopus, oyster, prawns, scallop, shrimp, squid
vegetables (including vegetable-like fruits)	artichoke, arugula, asparagus, beet, bok choy, broccoli, Brussels sprouts, cabbage, carrots, cauliflower, celeriac/celery root, celery, chicory, collard greens, cucumber, daikon, dandelion, endive, fiddlehead, fennel, Jerusalem artichoke, jicama, kohlrabi, kale, leek, lettuce, mushrooms, olives, onion, plantain, pumpkin, purslane, radicchio, radish, rhubarb, rutabaga, scallion, shallot, spinach, spring onion, sunchoke, swede, sweet potato, Swiss chard, taro, turnip, water chestnuts, watercress, yam, zucchini
sea vegetables	dulse, kombu, nori, sea kale, wakame
fruits	apple, apricot, avocado, banana, blackberry, blueberry, cherry, cranberry, date, fig, grapefruit, grapes, kiwi, kumquat, lemon, lime, mandarin, mango, melon, nectarine, orange, papaya, peach, pear, pineapple, plum, pomegranate, quince, raspberry, strawberry, watermelon
herbs and spices	basil, bay leaf, chamomile, chives, cilantro, cinnamon, cloves, dill weed, garlic, ginger, horseradish, kaffir lime, lavender, lemongrass, mace, marjoram, mint, oregano, parsley, rosemary, saffron, sage, tarragon, thyme, turmeric, vanilla bean, wasabi
ferments	beet kvass, coconut kefir/yogurt, kombucha, lacto-fermented fruits and vegetables, sauerkraut, water kefir
fats (check ingredients)	avocado oil, bacon grease, coconut oil, lard (pork), leaf lard, olive oil, palm oil, palm shortening, poultry fat, tallow (beef/lamb)
sweeteners (in moderation)	blackstrap molasses, coconut sugar, coconut syrup, honey, maple sugar, maple syrup
pantry	agar agar, arrowroot, baking soda, capers, carob, cassava, coconut products, fish sauce (check ingredients), gelatin, green banana flour, tapioca flour, vinegar (apple cider, balsamic, white/red wine)

FOODS TO AVOID

The "avoid" list may be a lengthy one, but there are plenty of delicious foods to eat. There are also new ones waiting to be discovered—perhaps even a new favorite. It's crucial to replace eliminated foods, so make it a challenge to seek out new produce to try. Additionally, our brain can be retrained if we repeat our thoughts enough: Don't spend time thinking of all the foods you cannot have; instead tell yourself about those that you *can* have. There are so many choices!

grains and pseudo-grains	amaranth, barley, buckwheat, bulgur, corn, couscous, durum, farro, Job's tears, kamut, millet, oat, quinoa, rice, rye, sorghum, spelt, teff, triticale, wheat, wild rice
dairy	butter, buttermilk, cheese, cottage cheese, cream, cream cheese, ghee, heavy cream, ice cream, kefir, milk, sour cream, whey, whipping cream, yogurt
eggs	chicken, duck, goose, quail, and all other types
nuts (including flours, butters, or oils derived from them)	almond, Brazil, cashew, chestnut, hazelnut, macadamia, pecan, pine nuts, pistachio, walnut
seeds (including flours, butters, spices or oils derived from them)	anise, caraway, celery seed, chia, chocolate, cocoa, coffee, coriander, cumin, dill seed, fennel seed, fenugreek, flax, hemp, mustard, nutmeg, pine nut, poppy, pumpkin, sesame, sunflower
legumes	adzuki bean, black bean, black-eyed pea, butter beans, cannellini bean, chickpea/garbanzo bean, fava bean, Great Northern bean, green bean, kidney bean, lentil, lima bean, mung bean, navy bean, pea, peanut, pinto bean, runner bean, snow peas, soybean (and products derived from soy), split peas, sugar snap peas
fats	canola oil, corn oil, cottonseed oil, olive oil (cold press), palm kernel oil, peanut oil, safflower oil, sunflower oil, soybean oil
nightshades (including spices derived from them)	ashwagandha, bell pepper, cayenne pepper, chili pepper, eggplant, goji berry, ground cherry, hot pepper, paprika, potato, tomatillo, tomato
fruit and berry spices	allspice, caraway, cardamom, juniper, pepper (black, white, green, pink), sumac, star anise
additional ingredients	alcohol, artificial coloring and flavoring, emulsifiers, nitrates and nitrites, nonnutritive sweeteners (including stevia), processed foods, refined sugars, stabilizers, sugar alcohols, thickeners

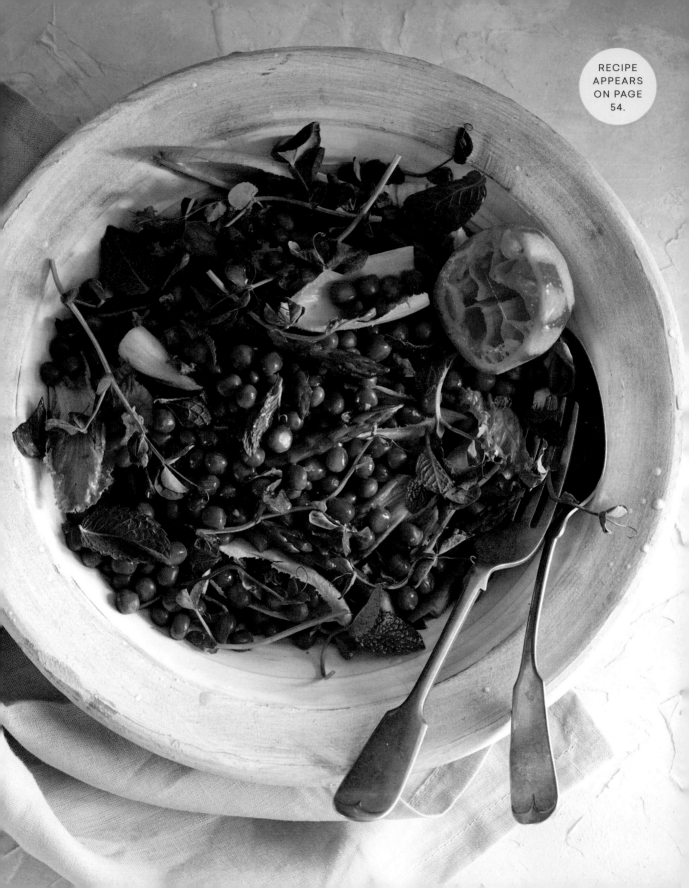

RECIPE APPEARS ON PAGE 54.

CHAPTER TWO

THE REINTRODUCTION PROCESS

YOU MAY THINK that people can't wait to transition off the strict elimination phase of the AIP. Often the opposite scenario happens. Some people are anxious about jeopardizing the healing they've gained during the elimination phase and want to stay there indefinitely. Others don't want to leave the comfort zone of arbitrary food lists and face decisions about which foods to reintroduce. Still others may not feel confident that they can recognize an adverse reaction and believe that staying in the initial phase is a safe bet. The thought of moving on to reintroductions might be scary; if this is you, believe me, you are not alone.

Reintroductions don't need to be a source of anxiety or trepidation. Take a moment to think about all the hard work you've put in so far. Recognize how far you have already come. In this chapter, you'll learn to gauge when the time is right for reintroduction, what to do, and how to go about it. What's more, this book is filled with delicious, nourishing meals to incorporate as you go through the process. Far from being something to dread, this is an exciting and empowering time. You are healing!

THE IMPORTANCE OF REINTRODUCING FOODS

There are several reasons why the reintroduction process matters for your healing and your body—and nutritional benefits are at the top of that list.

1. **Expand your diet to add interest.** When we eat the same foods day in and day out, we get bored and our body may suffer. Healing the gut is more challenging if we are lacking in nutrients, and there is more chance of developing further food sensitivities. But there is good news: Some new foods may even make you feel better, as they expand your nutrient stores.

> **Keep in mind that benefits will only be relevant if you tolerate the foods in question. If your immune system flags a food as an invader, it is anything but healthy.**
>
> **If you are not able to tolerate egg whites but can tolerate the yolks, be sure to include them (e.g., raw in mayonnaise, hard-boiled and crumbled over salads or soups, or used in your baking). Nuts and seeds are high in omega-6 though, so large amounts can increase inflammation. Soaking and sprouting, when possible, prior to eating will make them much more digestible.**

2. **A wider range of foods means a wider range of nutrients.** Despite kale, collards, and Swiss chard being similar dark leafy greens, they each contain different concentrations of nutrients. For example, kale is considerably higher in vitamin C than the others. Collards contain the most calcium, and Swiss chard the richest source of iron. These leaves are all elimination-phase compliant; however, there are rich pickings of essential nutrients from reintroduction foods, too. If you are able to eat yogurt from grass-fed cows, then your calcium intake gets a further boost. The same will happen to your vitamin C levels when you consume red bell pepper. When you tolerate pumpkin seeds you'll be getting a super-rich burst of zinc, and nuts such as almonds and hazelnuts supply a very decent amount of vitamin E. Whichever phase you are on, you should aim to consume as many different foods as you can, because what you are ultimately looking for is the least restricted diet possible.

3. **Add foods to gain significant health benefits.** Always keep in mind that reintroductions are also essential for your overall health. Eggs are a rich source of healthy protein, omega-3 fatty acids, and many vitamins and minerals. Nuts and seeds contain many essential micronutrients and are rich in healthy protein and fats. Grass-fed butter is a wonderfully rich source of nutrients, including fat-soluble vitamin K2 and butyric acid; not easily found in other foods, these are both important for pushing down inflammation. Other key nutrients are vitamins A and D, which are extremely important for gut healing.

4. **Reintroductions allow more food freedom.** Having some reintroductions in your arsenal will help enormously when it comes to visiting friends and family, dining out at restaurants or potlucks, attending work meetings and parties, and enjoying trips, vacations, and those moments of spontaneity. Even the addition of black pepper is going to broaden your food choices on a menu or at the deli counter. Reintroductions can also make it easier to cope with others who try to cajole you to eat foods that are on the avoid list (perhaps you've even experienced the "a little bit won't really hurt" mentality).

5. **Long delays may create food fear.** It's important to have your goals in sight, but it is not healthy to allow food choices to control life to the extent that enjoyment of eating and socializing is lost. If you experience feelings of depression, anxiety, or even paranoia about getting sick from eliminated foods, please reach out for professional advice, or to someone whom you feel comfortable confiding in, to help put some balance into your life.

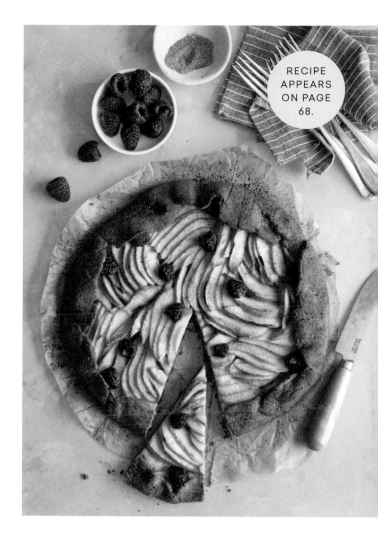

RECIPE APPEARS ON PAGE 68.

WHY REINTRODUCE IN STAGES?

Some people will start with reintroducing the foods they've missed the most, such as cheese or tomatoes. While this is completely understandable, the reintroduction stages laid out by Dr. Sarah Ballantyne offer the highest chance of success. Those foods listed in Stage 1 are typically the foods least likely to cause a reaction, because they are the least irritating to the gut and more nutrient dense. At the other extreme,

Stage 4 foods are the most likely offenders, so you would be wise to leave them until you have a good number of reintroductions under your belt, together with a significant amount of healing.

Concentrating on the most nutritious foods makes sense: The more nourished you are, the better your gut and immune health will be. This will bring a greater chance of success in the long run. So, if you've been pining for certain things,

REINTRODUCTION STAGES

Below are the Four Stages of Reintroduction. Foods listed in bold are featured in recipes in this book.

1

Egg Yolks	**All types**
Legumes (with edible pods/sprouts)	Green beans, **peas**, runner beans, snow peas, **sugar snap peas,**
Fruit and berry-based spices	**Allspice**, caraway, **cardamom**, **juniper**, **pepper** (black, green, pink, white), **star anise**, **sumac**
Seed-based spices	Anise, annatto, black caraway (Russian caraway, black cumin), celery seed, **coriander seed**, **cumin**, dill seed, **fennel seed**, fenugreek seed, **mustard**, **nutmeg**
Nuts and seed (oils only)	Macadamia, **sesame**, **walnut**
Nuts and seeds	**Chocolate**, cocoa, **cacao**, **coffee** (occasional basis)
Dairy (grass-fed)	**Ghee**

2

Nuts and seeds (including whole, ground, flours, butters, oils)	**Almonds**, Brazil nuts, **cashews**, **chestnuts**, **hazelnuts**, **macadamia nuts**, **pecans**, pine nuts, **pistachios**, **walnuts**, **chia**, **coffee** (daily basis), flax, **hemp**, **poppy**, pumpkin, sesame, **sunflower**
Egg whites (or whole eggs)	**All types**
Dairy (grass-fed)	**Butter** and butter oil
Alcohol (small quantities)	Fortified wine, gluten-free beer or hard cider, gluten-free spirits, **liqueur**, wine

3	Nightshades	**Bell (sweet) peppers**, **eggplant**, **paprika**, **peeled potatoes**
	Dairy (grass-fed)	**Buttermilk**, **cheese**, cottage cheese, cream, **cream cheese**, creme fraiche, curds, dairy-protein isolates, heavy cream, ice cream, **kefir**, **milk**, **sour cream**, whey, whey-protein isolate, **whipping cream**, **yogurt**
	Legumes (ideally soaked/fermented)	**Chickpeas** (garbanzo beans), **lentils**, **split peas**

4	Nightshades and their spices	Ashwaganda, cape gooseberries (ground cherries), **cayenne**, garden huckleberries, goji berries (wolfberries), **hot peppers** (chili etc), naranjillas, pepinos, pimentos, **unpeeled potatoes**, tomatillos, **tomatoes**
	Gluten-free grains, pseudo-grains (ideally soaked/fermented)	**Corn**, fonio, Job's tears, millet, **oats**, **rice**, sorghum, teff, **wild rice**, amaranth, **buckwheat**, quinoa
	Legumes	Adzuki beans, black beans, black-eyed peas, butter beans, calico beans, **cannellini beans**, fava beans (broad beans), **Great Northern beans**, Italian beans, kidney beans, lima beans, mung beans, navy beans, pinto beans, **peanuts**
	Alcohol (moderate quantities)	Gluten-free beer or hard cider, **wine**, fortified wine, **liqueur**, gluten-free spirits

you might choose to alternate between nutrient density and desire.

Always remember: All foods should be reintroduced one at a time. While allowing you to keep a good record of successful challenges, it is essential for identifying foods that may be difficult for you. When you know what food is causing you trouble, you can leave it aside and try it again later in the process.

Also keep in mind that in the case of unwanted weight loss and/or extreme fatigue, you may wish to put white rice further up the list to try as an occasional food choice. It is the grain that is most likely tolerated.

You may find certain foods consistently challenging to put back into your diet. For some, the nightshade family, including eggplants, white potatoes, tomatoes, and hot peppers, is a source of difficulty: These are high in lectin, saponin, and/or capsaicin, all natural chemicals known to increase gut permeability, and generally hard for those with joint issues such as rheumatoid arthritis to tolerate. Similarly, some or all dairy might cause issues because it contains varying levels of casein, a protein similar to gliadin, which is found in gluten. Don't rush these foods, and be sure to try them in the correct order.

As tempting as it is to hurry the process once started, do take your time rather than risking unnecessary flare-ups and inflammation that may ultimately see you taking several steps backward. Expect this to be a long process, but it is so worth taking slowly. As is often the way, take heed from the Aesop's tortoise mindset: "Slow and steady wins the race."

JOURNALING IS CRUCIAL

Using a food and mood journal is a useful tool in both the elimination and reintroduction phases of the AIP. Writing down this information is a highly effective way of identifying why you may be having symptoms. Since reactions can take several days to appear, it can be easy to forget when they appeared and perhaps whether they even occurred at all. Keeping a daily log enables you to look back through your journals and, over time, you should begin to see a correlation between what you're consuming and how you feel in the hours and days that follow.

Logging your sleep pattern is also important. I know from personal experience that a restless night may set me up for a gut-tender day. Over time, my journal may help me figure out why I had that bad night in the first place. Documenting your exercise output, together with water intake, will help you track whether symptoms are related to over-strenuous (or lack of) activity, or hydration issues. Noting medications and/or supplements you are taking is recommended; they often contain fillers to which people with autoimmune disease may react badly. They also may contain stimulating ingredients that are ramping up your immune system.

In short, when it comes to tracking your success with reintroductions, journaling gives you a reliable reference to help you stay on track in reaching your goals. If you document your progress on a scale of 1 to 10, where 1 indicates not great at all and 10 means fantastic, you'll find it much more informative than jotting down whether you've had a "good" or "bad" day. A numeric scale more precisely conveys the severity (or not) of symptoms.

If you find that journaling is causing anxiety or obsessive behavior, it is highly recommended that you reach out to a practitioner who can help you reach your health goals.

PREPARING FOR SUCCESS

As with the elimination phase of the protocol, you are still a work in progress. To have arrived at the reintroduction stage means you've already put in a lot of work and are healing. Use that same commitment with this next stage to ensure you reap rewards. It is crucial to put yourself at the top of your list of priorities and continue working on your lifestyle. How you deal with sleep and stress management can quickly affect your gut microbiome, for better or worse. Good digestion enables your body to absorb the nutrients required to keep you in balance. Movement, fresh air, social connection, and finding joy in life will ensure you are on the right path.

Gut healing is an essential part of the elimination phase, and it should be carried on throughout the reintroduction phase. So keep focusing on nourishing your body with high-nutrient foods such as organ meat, shellfish, seafood, and sea vegetables, herbs and other leafy greens, colorful vegetables, bone broth, and fermented foods. Minimize the baked goods and other treats; they may fill you up, but they lack higher levels of nutrition. Feed your microbiome with the foods mentioned on page 30-31. Variety is key to packing in as wide a range of vitamins, minerals, phytonutrients, and essential fiber as possible.

Support your liver, which is your main detoxification organ. Eat beets and bitter leaves, drink dandelion tea, use a castor oil pack at night, or at least rub a couple of teaspoons of castor oil into the liver area, which is on the right side of the rib cage underneath the breast.

Do dry skin brushing each morning before stepping into a warm shower. This stimulates the lymphatic system to release toxins, as well as exfoliates dead skin cells to improve detox pathways. Using a medium-soft bristle brush and a light touch, gently work from the feet and hands upward toward the heart. Lightly brush in a clockwise circular motion around the belly and be particularly gentle over delicate areas such as the breasts and groin.

Regulate your circadian rhythms with quality sleep, or try napping in the event that's not possible. Wear amber-tinted glasses for two or three hours leading up to bedtime. Set a nighttime routine and stick to it. See more on this on page 21-22.

Don't make any other changes as you go through each food reintroduction. If you start a new workout or dance routine at the same time, for example, you won't know whether any reaction is down to the food you are challenging or the lifestyle change. Similarly, if your doctor has put you on a new medicine or supplement, allow a sensible "honeymoon" period before attempting a food reintroduction.

Become tuned in to your body so you have a greater chance of identifying a reaction sooner than later. Check out the free audio body scan on my blog. Above all, develop a mindset of success rather than failure. You absolutely can do this!

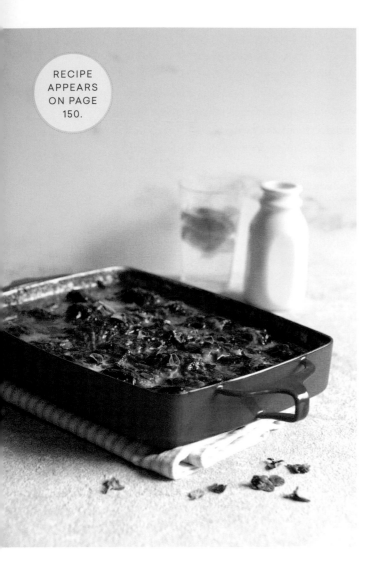

RECIPE APPEARS ON PAGE 150.

but the reality is most people should wait for sixty to ninety days, perhaps longer. You need to see enough improvement in your symptoms to give you a measure against which you can test any reactions. This measure is your barometer of wellness.

There's no need to rush this process, so don't get out your calendar and decide on a start date just yet. Your journal will be invaluable here. We tend to get so used to how we feel on a day-to-day basis that our improvements are overlooked. When you review your notes, you will realize what a long way you have come.

YOU DON'T NEED TO BE IN COMPLETE REMISSION

Although the ideal, not everyone will see complete remission, possibly due to long-term tissue or organ damage. Also, autoimmune diseases often present themselves differently, so some people may be symptomatic for quite a while. You may always require medication, for example, so this is where monitoring regular blood work will come in handy as a way to assess your progress.

It is crucial that you are able to recognize a reaction should you have one. The last thing you want is several reintroductions under your belt, only to find you are having symptoms further down the line and no clue what caused them. In this instance you may find it quicker and less stressful to go back to the elimination phase, reset, and start the process over. As long as you have spent at least thirty days on the

KNOWING WHEN YOU ARE READY

Only you truly know when you are ready for reintroduction, but you should aim to stay on the elimination phase for a minimum of thirty days before considering reintroductions. You should start to see some improvements within this time,

strict elimination phase, achieved a stable and consistent measure of health, and seen positive changes in your digestion, skin, mood, sleep, energy, stress levels, and so on, you are good to go.

WHEN IT ISN'T A GOOD TIME

It's sensible to put yourself in a calm, familiar surrounding when you try a reintroduction. Going on vacation, dining out, or eating at someone else's home are not good times. After all, you want to be certain that any reaction experienced is related to food, rather than cross contamination or any other external factors you have unknowingly encountered.

It's also important to reintroduce food at a time when you are set up for success. Avoid added pressures such as a particularly busy period at work, if you are lacking in sleep or are sick, or at any other times of physical or emotional stress. If you are dealing with environmental allergies such as pollens or mold exposure, you would be wise to address those first. If you have weather-related symptoms, such as pressure headaches or mood issues, wait for the weather to settle first. If you are starting a new medication or supplement, be sure they are working well for you. If you have had a recent vaccination, do not choose this time to challenge your immune system still further.

You should never try to reintroduce anything to which you have a severe allergy, because this may put you into a flare and set you back several steps in your healing.

HOW TO ATTEMPT A REINTRODUCTION

Remember to introduce only one food at a time, and don't rush the process. Reintroducing too quickly may cause a flare. As you go through each food challenge, be honest with yourself about how you truly feel, not how you want to feel. It can be quite stress-inducing when there's something you want to eat so badly, but try your hardest to relax. If you notice your pulse quicken at the thought of trying a new food, do the breathing exercise on page 19.

When you are working your way through the reintroduction stages, there's no need to do every single food on the list before moving on to the next stage. Concentrate on the ones you want to eat and resist the temptation to have too much, too fast. Now choose a time when you're not feeling rushed, have your journal in hand, and document your progress in line with the steps below, as laid out by Dr. Sarah Ballantyne in her book *The Paleo Approach*.

7-step reintroduction challenge

1. Select a food to challenge. It can be raw or cooked. Note the date and food in your journal, including how you feel using the numeric scale of 1 to 10 (see page 32).

2. Eat ½ teaspoon or less (a nibble) and wait fifteen minutes. If you have symptoms, make a note and stop the challenge.

3. If there are no symptoms, eat 1 teaspoon of the food (tiny bite) and wait fifteen minutes. If you have symptoms, make a note and stop the challenge.

4. If there are no symptoms, eat 1½ teaspoons (slightly bigger bite) and wait two to three hours. If you have symptoms, make a note and stop the challenge.

5. If there are no symptoms, eat a normal-size portion of the food, either by itself or as part of a meal and wait three to seven days (five to seven is even better). Do not eat that food or reintroduce any others during this time and continue to journal. Make a note of any symptoms that occur.

6. If you have any symptoms during this time, do not include this food in your diet. Always wait until you get back to your numeric measure of health before trying a different food.

7. If there are no symptoms, you may bring this food back into your diet and select a new food to challenge.

When it comes to testing seed- and berry-based spices in Stage 1, eat these as you would normally, in other words included in a recipe. Follow the above steps by eating small amounts of your meal and freeze the remainder if necessary.

Once you are sure you have successfully reintroduced a food, don't then eat it on a daily basis. You don't want to develop a sensitivity to it. If you are still not too sure whether something is successful, make a note in your journal and leave this food out of your diet for a month or so. Once you are back to your original numeric measure, simply try another food. If there are any AIP-compliant foods that you don't tolerate well, treat them as you would potential future reintroductions.

It is highly recommended that you do not try to reintroduce gluten, because its immune response can last up to six months each time you eat it and is known to be highly damaging to the gut.

OCCASIONAL REINTRODUCTIONS: WHEN A FOOD ISN'T FOR EVERYDAY CONSUMPTION

When you go through the process, you may find that your body is only happy to tolerate one or more foods a couple of times a week. If this is the case, don't give up on this food, or push it more frequently. Respect your body and, for the next few months, incorporate it once or twice a week only. Over time you may find you can include it more frequently.

IDENTIFYING A REACTION

Unfortunately, a reaction can come in many forms, at any time. It could resemble the return of your previous symptoms or something completely new.

Signs of a reaction may include any of the following:

- Digestive changes: bloating, gas, belching, abdominal pain/cramping, nausea, diarrhea, constipation, anal itching, hemorrhoids, undigested food in stool, changes in bowel movements (including timing), heartburn, acid reflux, gurgling in the throat

- Sleep difficulties: unable to stay awake, unable to fall asleep, waking in the night, not feeling rested in the morning

- Cravings: for sugar, fat, caffeine, nonfood items such as clay, chalk, dirt
- Skin irritations: rashes, swelling/redness, acne/pimples, pink bumps or spots, hives, eczema, itchy/dry skin, dry hair/nails
- Aches/pains/stiffness: areas affected may include muscles, joints, tendons, ligaments
- Mood changes: mood swings, depression, unable to deal with stress, increased anxiety, over emotional, easily upset
- Energy fluctuation: reduced energy, fatigue, sleepy in the afternoon, wired at night
- Other symptoms: headaches/migraines, dizzy or lightheaded, brain fog, poor concentration, tinnitus, blocked ears, sinus congestion, phlegm/runny nose/postnasal drip, coughing/wheezing, increased need to clear throat, mouth ulcers, itchy eyes/mouth/nose/ears, sneezing, return or worsening of symptoms, racing pulse

One person's symptoms may be different from another's. Some reactions may show up fairly quickly, perhaps even before you have finished your meal. Other reactions are cumulative and may appear up to several days later, typically in the case of skin reactions. If you are concerned about whether you'll know a reaction if it occurs, check out the free audio body scan on my blog (see Resources, page 202), which is designed to help cultivate awareness of your body.

Any time you have suspicions about whether you are tolerating a food, use the mantra "If in doubt, leave it out!" You can always try again in the future.

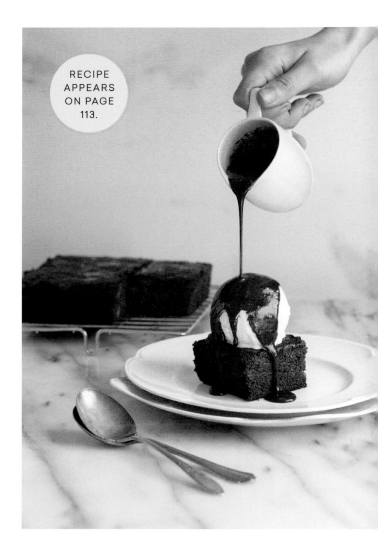

RECIPE APPEARS ON PAGE 113.

REACTIONS IN CHILDREN

Children are usually less in tune with their bodies or unable/unwilling to articulate a problem. You might not notice skin rashes if they are covered by clothing. They may not want to tell you about any symptoms after eating a favorite food, for fear you'll take it away. In these cases, be aware of anything out of character, such as disrupted sleep, bed wetting, changes in bowel movements, or emotional or behavioral changes. Write a note to try the suspected food at another time and, if the same thing occurs, mark it as a reaction.

DEALING WITH AN UNSUCCESSFUL ATTEMPT

First, don't allow yourself to be put off, or lose faith in the process. Remember: Just because one food attempt was unsuccessful doesn't mean others will be. Trust your body's ability to heal, but remember this can take time.

If you have a reaction, make a note in your journal and stop trying to reintroduce that particular food for the time being. If it's a slight reaction, concentrate on nourishing yourself with nutrient-dense foods and wait until you get back to your original numeric measure before attempting something new. If you have a significant reaction, put all future reintroduction attempts on hold, go back to the elimination phase, and manage your

flare as outlined on page 39. It's impossible to say how long you should wait before attempting your next reintroduction: It could be days, weeks, or longer. Listen to your body. You will know when the time is right.

how to restart reintroductions

1. When it's time to restart, you shouldn't need to go right back to the beginning. Pick a new food and continue as before, being vigilant about any reactions. As for the food that caused the flare-up, do not attempt to reintroduce that one for some time. Be aware that there's a possibility it might never be tolerated.

2. If you are unsuccessful with one food from Stage 1, try some more in that section and see whether they are tolerated. If not, your body is telling you it needs more healing and you should return to the elimination phase.

3. If you have made several reintroductions already, skip the one that hasn't worked and try something else. Move on to Stage 2 when you feel ready. You can reattempt the original food in the future.

4. Finally, before putting the blame on a particular food, reread your journal to be clear about what else has happened over the preceding days. Check whether there's some improvement you can make on your lifestyle.

Above all, try and put a positive spin on any unsuccessful reintroduction. You are not a failure. This may sound like an odd thing to say, but the amazing thing here is that your body is able to communicate this with you. How awesome is that?

WHAT IS EFT?

EFT, also known as tapping, is a needleless acupressure technique performed by gently tapping on meridian points on the upper body, to support emotional health. It is particularly effective as a holistic way to manage pain, stress, and anxiety. To learn more, see Resources on page 202.

HOW TO MANAGE A FLARE-UP OF SYMPTOMS (OR NEW ONES)

A flare-up can be a major disappointment. It's important to listen to your body: It is telling you something. Take the time to slow down. Then, try these strategies to address the flare-up:

- Go back to the strict AIP until you are in control of your symptoms and back to your original numeric measure of health.

- Optimize sleep, taking short naps if necessary.

- Assess your levels of activity, whether it be too much or too little.

- Make sure you are properly hydrated by drinking plenty of pure, filtered water.

- Seek out connections with people and things that make you happy.

- Find a love for life and acceptance of your reality.

- Step up your intake of nutrient-dense foods.

Next, incorporate extra self-care such as EFT (Emotional Freedom Technique, or tapping) to manage pain and anxiety. Meditation, yoga, and gentle stretching will refocus you. Avoiding the news will reduce emotional stress. Journaling and a coloring book will ground you. A hot Epsom salt bath complete with essential oils, candles, soft music, and a face pack will relax and help you sleep well. A gentle massage, such as lymphatic drainage, will help move toxins along.

Finding an empathetic community will uplift and empower you.

The AIP community is a growing and supportive one. You will find many online forums; some may even be local to you. These are great options for seeking support from people who understand what you're going through. If you prefer to stay offline, look for local meet-up groups, or start one yourself. You won't be the only person in need of a friendly face or two to share experiences.

THE IMPORTANCE OF CONTINUED NUTRIENT DENSITY AND SELF-CARE

You should always have your sights on nutrient density. We are made up of 100 trillion cells, each one relying on quality nutrients to supply the energy that builds new cells and tissues, which in turn make up our organs. These cells need proper fuel to release waste, repair and rebuild, and ultimately keep us safe from dysfunction, degeneration, and disease.

Because our cells are working nonstop, you can see why they are going to need all the help they can get—that's where self-care comes into play. The lifestyle component is essential and ongoing. Quality sleep is critical for decreasing inflammation, but many people don't get anywhere near enough. Detoxification, repair, regeneration, and myriad other incredible functions happen while we sleep, which is why it's recommended to be in bed no later than 10 p.m. We should be aiming for eight to ten hours each night, with an absolute minimum of seven hours.

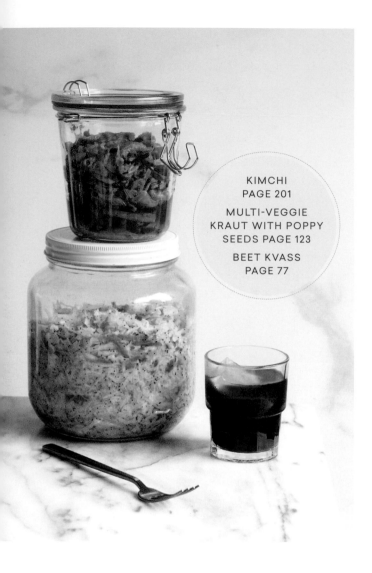

KIMCHI
PAGE 201

MULTI-VEGGIE
KRAUT WITH POPPY
SEEDS PAGE 123

BEET KVASS
PAGE 77

by stimulating acupressure points throughout the back to activate a deep relaxation response. When you stick to a routine, your body will soon behave like one of Pavlov's dogs and know when it's time to wind down for a good night's sleep.

Aim to finish your last meal at least two hours before bed, preferably three, so that digestion can take place before you go to sleep. If you eat too late, your body will prioritize digestion while you're sleeping, at the expense of everything else. If you feel wired at night, avoid screens and electronics at least one hour before bed and try wearing blue light–blocking glasses as soon as the sun goes down. They don't look particularly stylish, but together with sleeping in a dark, relatively cool room and getting outside into the light first thing in the morning, they will help to reset your circadian rhythms.

Managing stress is crucial for optimal health, especially when you are dealing with auto-immune disease. Every day we need to make choices about what is important, and finding that balance is often hard to do. Incorporate some downtime, get out into nature, and find content-ment whenever and wherever possible. Rather than seeing self-care as indulgent, recognize the positive benefits of shifting your thinking to "going without is not an option."

Movement is another necessary element that falls under the self-care umbrella. Unlike high-in-tensity training, which is stressful on the gut, low-intensity activity will help decrease inflam-mation. Do whatever you feel capable of without pushing yourself too hard. If you're not particu-larly mobile, don't worry: A gentle walk outside is progress. Daily activity will help to regulate hormones and inflammation, as well as allow the lymphatic system to move freely and detoxify.

If quality sleep seems unobtainable to you, try getting into a nightly routine such as a hot bath with Epsom salts and a calming essential oil, a mug of chamomile tea, followed by a meditation or body scan (see Resources, page 202, for a free download). Perhaps spend time applying your facial products as you do some light breath work. I like my sleep induction mat, which works

You will also achieve improved sleep, better mood, and more successful stress management. And if you aren't mobile at all, the benefits of being outside and just getting some fresh air are still huge.

Lastly, we are social beings, therefore we need to make time to be with others as often as possible. Laughter is truly a powerful medicine, so choose to be with those who light you up rather than rob your energy. As Dr. James L. Wilson describes in his book *Adrenal Fatigue: The 21st Century Stress Syndrome*, "energy robbers are like holes in the barrel preventing you from being full of energy."

WHY YOU MAY BE HAVING TROUBLE REINTRODUCING FOODS

If you run into difficulties during reintroduction, I want to reiterate you are *not* a failure. Please don't be put off, throw in the towel, or lose faith in the process. Trust in your amazing body's desire and ability to heal.

If you are unsure whether a reintroduction is working, or have made some reintroductions but not others in the same stage, it's worth doing some investigating. Think about these possible scenarios:

- Some people find they can tolerate certain foods better if they are either raw or cooked, so try both when possible.

- If you cannot introduce black pepper, try white pepper instead. They are from the same plant but have been processed differently. Black pepper is picked while unripe and then dried. White pepper is from fully ripe berries that have been soaked or rinsed to remove the skins.

- Oats are naturally gluten-free, but they are typically processed in a plant that has wheat or other gluten-containing grains. You may have better luck with certified gluten-free oats.

- Nuts such as cashews, seeds such as coffee, and peanuts (legumes) are all linked with mold issues. If you notice consistent difficulties reintroducing these foods, mold could be a problem and further investigation may be warranted.

- If you are having problems reintroducing nuts and seeds, be sure you are soaking, sprouting, and dehydrating them, where relevant. This will make them easier to digest and you may have more success. Soaking and pressure-cooking legumes significantly reduces antinutrients, making them more easily digestible. See pages 11–12 of Kitchen Basics.

- Dairy differs depending on the amount of milk proteins; it's not unusual for people to tolerate some but not others. Start by reintroducing ghee. If you cannot reintroduce ghee, don't try to reintroduce any other dairy products. If ghee is well tolerated, try butter and then other dairy products, bearing in mind goat dairy is easier to tolerate than cow. Aim for grass-fed, preferably raw, for a higher chance of success, and always reintroduce separately. Try A2 milk, which is easier to digest because it contains only one beta-casein protein.

- If you're having problems with chicken eggs, source duck, goose, or quail eggs instead. Try the yolks cooked (hard-boil and separate the yolk from the white, discarding the membrane) and raw. Are you buying eggs from birds that have been allowed to roam outside, foraging plants and insects, free from hormones and antibiotics? If eggs are still not successful, look at what the birds have been fed. Most are fed soy, so search for soy-free eggs. You never know—it could be the feed you're reacting to and not the eggs after all.

If you cannot bring in any reintroductions at all (or very few), ask yourself the following questions:

- How long have you spent on the elimination phase? Thirty days is too short for most people to see enough improvements.

- Are you absolutely certain you have been following the elimination phase properly and not eating something that should have been avoided?

- Are you prioritizing foods that are high in nutrients and keeping treats to the minimum?

- Are you eating organic produce or following the Dirty Dozen/Clean Fifteen lists (see Resources, page 202)?

- Are you buying grass-fed but grain-finished meat? Many grass-fed cows are finished with barley during the final few months. Or are you not buying grass-fed meat at all? In both cases you may be sensitive to the grain feed.

- Are you buying wild-caught fish, rather than farmed? Farmed fish are fed a range of foods such as feathers and grains, and given antibiotics, which may be causing inflammation.

- Is it possible you are getting gluten exposure on a frequent basis? Maybe from other family members, your roommates, or your local café?

- Did you begin your reintroduction with the Stage 1 foods that are typically less irritating to the gut? Or did you skip ahead to something on the Stage 4 list, for example?

- Are you including self-care in your day? Do you have effective methods to manage stress? Are you getting enough sleep and gentle movement, and are you seeking joy?

If you can relate to any of the above, go back to the strict elimination phase with a focus on eating nutrient-dense foods. Don't worry: You can always try reintroductions again after thirty days on the elimination phase.

WHEN YOU NEED TO TROUBLESHOOT

If after three to four months you're not making the progress you had hoped for, it's time to troubleshoot. Be sure you've been doing the protocol correctly, and seek the help of someone who can guide you through the next step. AIP Certified Coaches have been specifically trained for this purpose. Finding a medical practitioner who is knowledgeable in the AIP may be harder but is certainly worth the search.

In the event you have reached a plateau, are becoming more symptomatic, or are not able to reintroduce any foods, look deeper for reasons why your healing is compromised. It could be that you have underlying viral, bacterial, yeast, or parasite infections. *H. pylori* or small intestinal bacterial overgrowth (SIBO) are very common. Other factors such as blood sugar imbalance, poor methylation, histamine intolerance, or mold toxicity could be blocking your progress, and these can all be unearthed by a skilled practitioner through appropriate testing. If you have unhealed trauma, post-traumatic stress disorder (PTSD), stress eating, or addiction, these emotional and psychological issues could be the missing link in your recovery.

IN THE MEDICINE CABINET

I like to have the following digestive supplements on hand:

Digestive enzymes: These break down foods so that they can be more easily absorbed. Very useful for optimizing digestion, they can be beneficial when eating out. As ever, it's best to consult your practitioner to see whether they will be good for you, and check ingredients carefully, as corn and soy are very often used as fillers in supplements. Do not introduce these at the same time as you are introducing a new food.

Activated charcoal: This is great to have in the cabinet at all times because it binds and eliminates food from the GI tract sooner than later. It's really helpful for times when you have food poisoning, been "glutened," or have digestive issues brought on by food. It also makes a great face mask! Do not use on a regular basis, though, because it also removes nutrients.

BEFORE YOU START REINTRODUCTIONS

Lay some strong foundations to set yourself up for success: Optimize your digestion (page 19). When you are digesting efficiently, you'll absorb more nutrients and your immune system becomes stronger.

Do the breathing exercise on page 19. Once you feel that shift, put a forkful of food into your mouth and chew like you've probably never chewed before. Include bitter leaves, beets, dandelion leaves, broccoli sprouts, and cruciferous veggies in your meals. These foods help to unburden the liver, which, as you know, is your main detoxification organ. You'll find these in recipes throughout this book.

If you need inner support, write out an intention card to remind you of your goals and priorities. Write a few lines of gratitude that you've found this amazing protocol and a supportive community, and that you're empowering yourself by advocating for your own health. Have patience in the process. You *are* healing!

READY TO START?

If you follow the process with small actionable steps, you are far less likely to cause a flare. Know that there will likely be hiccups along the way, and that's not the end of the world. Try to enjoy the process. Congratulate yourself on each and every one of your successes. Sending you much luck!

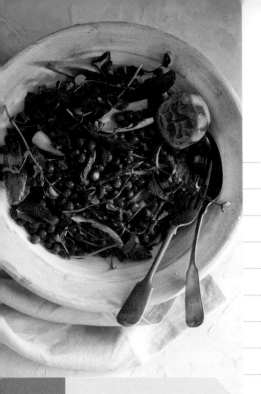

STAGE 1 RECIPES

RECIPE APPEARS ON PAGE 54.

CHAPTER THREE

STAGE 1 RECIPES

WELCOME TO THE START of a new chapter—literally and metaphorically. I hope you're excited about the possibilities that lie ahead. You're about to begin a renewed relationship with foods you haven't eaten in a long while. This first stage is where you'll be introducing some key nutrients and flavors, and as you progress you will be building your future maintenance template.

If you've started the reintroduction process, you'll find plenty of recipes to incorporate new foods. If you're still on the elimination phase, nearly all the recipes can be tweaked without losing out on flavor. And if you're just here for the recipes—a feast awaits!

Egg yolks are one of the most nutrient-dense foods on the planet and should be among the first reintroductions you attempt. Crumble cooked yolks over salads and skillet meals, mix them into burgers and meatballs, or add them to sauces. And you will get the maximum experience from freshly made Mint Mayonnaise (page 81) and melt-in-your-mouth Mini Custard Tarts (page 72).

Another important reintroduction is ghee (clarified butter), ideally from grass-fed sources. Ghee is your gateway to reintroducing dairy, and is used here as both a cooking fat and baking ingredient.

Spices rubbed onto meat, fish, and vegetables before roasting are always a winner to my mind. One of my favorite spices is cardamom, and it's especially lovely in the rustic Pear, Raspberry, and Cardamom Galette (page 68) in this chapter. A spice I know a lot of people miss is mustard. So, you can spoon Windfall Country Mustard (page 79) directly onto your plate or incorporate into the cauli rice that accompanies New York steak (page 66).

Everybody needs a condiment for an instant pep. I grew up with a bottle of brown sauce on the table whenever fries made an appearance, and it's fair to say my life changed on the day I tried the version you'll find in this chapter (page 80).

Dried legumes will come later in the reintroduction phases, but now's your chance to be reunited with those with edible pods. The Broth-Braised Peas with Mint (page 54) embody summertime for me, even when eaten on a cold night in the middle of winter.

For many, the biggest wins in this first stage will be chocolate and coffee (occasional basis). If these foods get you excited, you'll love the antioxidant-rich Chocolate Sweet Potato Mud Cake (page 71) and the Coffee Berry Compote (page 76).

NO OATS OATMEAL
WITH BLUEBERRIES & NUTMEG

SERVES 4

PREP TIME:
15 MINUTES

COOK TIME:
10 MINUTES

OATMEAL

3 cups (765 g) precooked spaghetti squash

1¼ cups (120 g) shredded coconut

2 cups (500 ml) coconut milk

1 small ripe banana, mashed

Pinch sea salt

COMPOTE

2 cups (310 g) frozen blueberries

1 teaspoon ground cinnamon

2–3 fresh gratings of nutmeg

Pinch ground cloves

2 teaspoons (10 ml) maple syrup

Pinch sea salt

▬▬▬ I've been experimenting with oatmeal look-a-likes for years and, believe me, once you have the basic template you can't go wrong. If you're new to the idea of squash as a substitute for oats, give it a try and you'll be a convert. It has a neutral flavor, plus the texture is just right. The compote can be made ahead of time and served reheated or cold. It also makes a delicious topping for yogurt or ice cream.

To make the oatmeal, put the squash, coconut, coconut milk, banana, and salt in a large pan. Add ½ cup (235 ml) water, mix well, and bring to a boil. Immediately turn down to a simmer and cook, stirring frequently until piping hot.

To make the compote, put the blueberries, cinnamon, nutmeg, cloves, maple syrup, and salt in a small pan. Add 2 teaspoons (10 ml) water and mix well. Put over low heat and cover the pan. Cook for 6 minutes, or until the blueberries are beginning to release their juices while retaining their shape. The liquid should be syrupy.

Remove the oatmeal from the heat. Using an immersion blender or a food processor, pulse briefly to break down the fibers of the squash while leaving it fairly chunky. Ladle the oatmeal into bowls and spoon over the compote. Serve immediately.

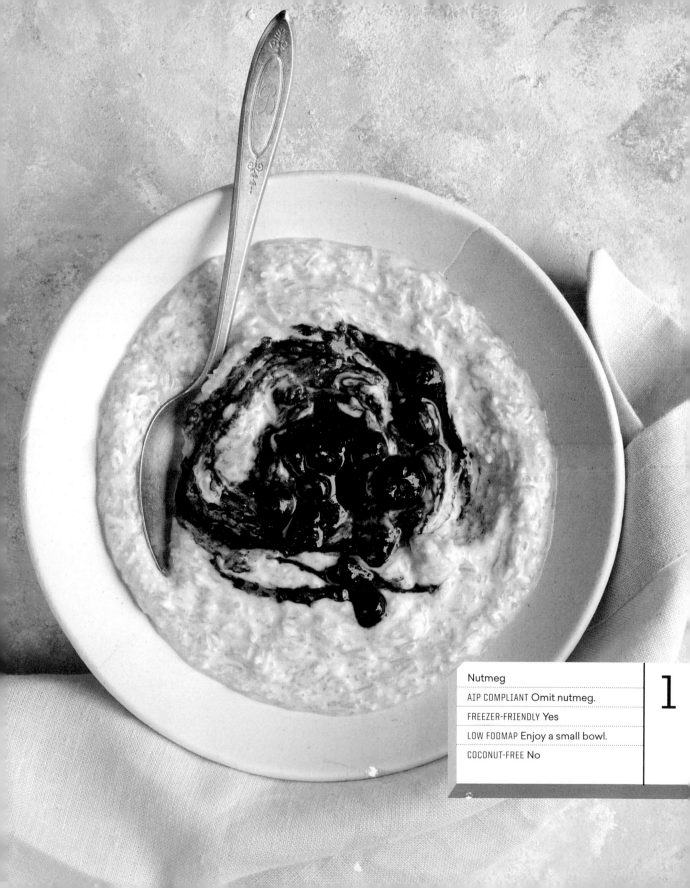

Nutmeg

AIP COMPLIANT Omit nutmeg.

FREEZER-FRIENDLY Yes

LOW FODMAP Enjoy a small bowl.

COCONUT-FREE No

1

BREAKFAST SKILLET

SERVES 5 TO 6

PREP TIME:
15 MINUTES

COOK TIME:
10 MINUTES

2 tablespoons (30 ml) extra virgin olive oil

1 lb (450 g) ground bison

10 oz (280 g) red cabbage, shredded

2 medium carrots, grated

1 small leek, shredded

3-inch (7.5 cm) piece daikon, grated

12 oz (340 g) rutabaga, grated

4 tablespoons (60 ml) coconut aminos

Pinch sea salt

Pinch black pepper

1 cup (60 g) roughly chopped fresh flat-leaf parsley

▬▬▬▬ I start most days with a breakfast skillet. It's a well-balanced macronutrient meal, and it's a great way to boost your rainbow veggie intake. This recipe has a good combination of sulfur-rich cruciferous vegetables, roots and leafy greens. Use this recipe as your template: Include anything that you have on hand or that needs using up. The cooking time depends on your preference. If your digestion is particularly compromised, cook the vegetables well. If you prefer them less cooked, adjust the timing accordingly.

Put a large sauté pan or skillet over medium heat and add the olive oil. Add the bison and cook for 4 minutes, or until browned.

Add the cabbage, carrots, leek, daikon, and rutabaga. Sauté for 5 to 8 minutes until tender, regulating the temperature if necessary. Stir in the coconut aminos, and add salt and pepper to taste.

Remove from the heat and stir in the parsley. Serve immediately.

1

Black pepper

AIP COMPLIANT Omit black pepper.

FREEZER-FRIENDLY Yes

LOW FODMAP Caution with coconut aminos.

COCONUT-FREE Omit coconut aminos.

HERBY
MUSHROOM SOUP

SERVES 4
PREP TIME: 20 MINUTES
COOK TIME: 35 MINUTES

1 tablespoon (14 g) ghee

6 oz (170 g) shallots, chopped

3 medium stalks celery, chopped

2 tablespoons (30 ml) olive oil

2 large cloves garlic, minced

12 oz (340 g) brown mushrooms, chopped

4 oz (110 g) white button mushrooms, chopped

4 oz (110 g) shiitake mushrooms, chopped

1 teaspoon finely chopped fresh rosemary

2 large sprigs fresh thyme

Pinch sea salt

Pinch black pepper (optional)

2 tablespoons (30 ml) sherry vinegar

5 cups (1.2 L) rich beef bone broth

2 cups (120 g) roughly chopped fresh flat-leaf parsley

1 cup (64 g) roughly chopped fresh dill

TO SERVE

¼ cup (60 g) coconut cream or yogurt

¼ cup (12 g) chopped chives

This is a creamy, nutritious soup with three different mushrooms—and a tasty treat for you and your microbiome. Here you can choose to include black pepper and/or ghee: The pepper adds a spicy kick to the soup. Ghee will enrichen it and add extra fat-soluble nutrients. Dr. Sarah Ballantyne has written extensively on the benefits of fungi, even elevating them to their own essential food group. So, dig in!

Heat the ghee in a large pan and add the shallots. Sauté over low heat for 5 to 6 minutes, or until softened. Add the celery and cook for 3 minutes. Add the oil with the garlic, mushrooms, rosemary, thyme, salt, and black pepper (if using).

Raise the heat to medium and continue cooking for 8 to 10 minutes, stirring frequently, until the mushrooms soften and release some of their juices.

Pour in the sherry vinegar. Scrape the sediment off the base of the pan and incorporate this into the mushroom mixture to add flavor to the soup. Pour in the broth and bring to a simmer. Cover and simmer for 10 minutes.

Remove the pan from the heat and add the parsley and dill. Allow to sit for 1 to 2 minutes until wilted. Discard the thyme sprigs. Transfer the soup to a blender and blitz until smooth. You will need to do this carefully in batches or use an immersion blender. Taste and adjust the seasoning if needed.

To serve, ladle into bowls, add a swirl of coconut cream together with a good pinch of chives.

Black pepper and/or ghee	
AIP COMPLIANT Sub extra virgin olive oil or other fat for ghee.	1
FREEZER-FRIENDLY Yes	
LOW FODMAP No	
COCONUT-FREE Omit cream swirl.	

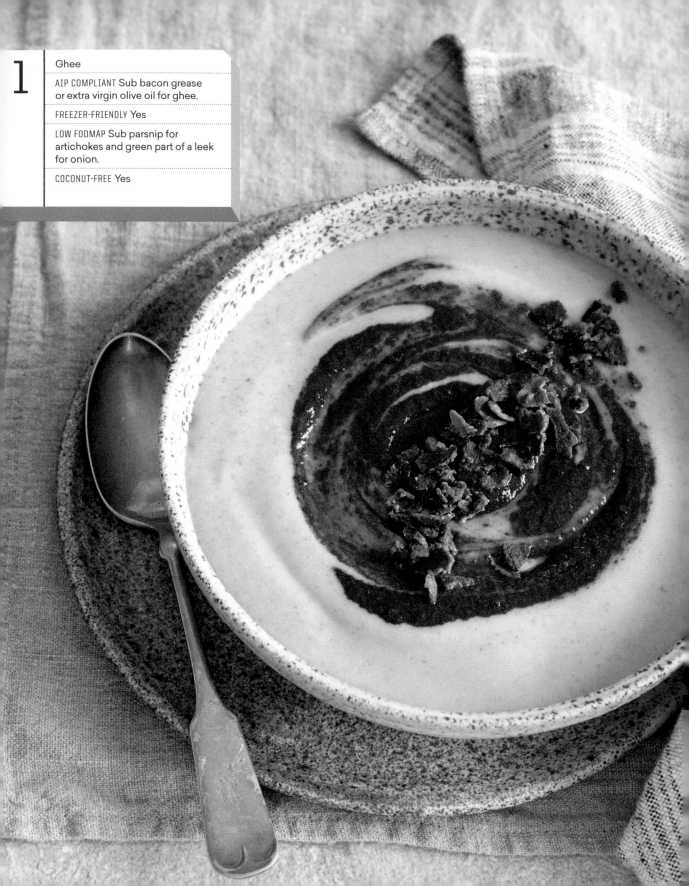

1 | Ghee

AIP COMPLIANT Sub bacon grease or extra virgin olive oil for ghee.

FREEZER-FRIENDLY Yes

LOW FODMAP Sub parsnip for artichokes and green part of a leek for onion.

COCONUT-FREE Yes

JERUSALEM ARTICHOKE SOUP
WITH CRUMBLED BACON

SERVES 4 TO 6

PREP TIME:
40 MINUTES

COOK TIME:
20 MINUTES

SOUP

1 tablespoon (14 g) ghee

1 medium onion,
finely chopped

1 tablespoon (15 ml)
lime juice

2 pounds (900 g)
Jerusalem artichokes
(sunchokes)

6 cups (1.4 L) chicken broth

Pinch sea salt

CRUMBLES

6 slices bacon

LEAFY SWIRL

2 large green kale leaves,
central stalk discarded

1½ cups (90 g) roughly
chopped fresh flat-leaf
parsley

½ cup plus 2 tablespoons
(155 ml) extra virgin
olive oil

1 tablespoon (15 ml)
lime juice

Pinch sea salt

This is a lovely smooth soup topped with a swirl of dark leafy greens and crunchy bacon. Jerusalem artichokes, also known as sunchokes, are a great source of resistant starch, which is important for feeding the beneficial bacteria living in your large intestine. If this is your first time eating Jerusalem artichokes, start with a small portion; not everyone finds them easy to digest. They're well worth trying though, both for their delicious flavor and for adding variety to your veggie repertoire.

To make the soup, heat the ghee in a large pan and add the onion. Sauté over gentle heat for 6 minutes until softened.

Fill a large bowl with water and add the lime juice. Scrub the Jerusalem artichokes and slice into ¼-inch (6-mm) rounds. As you do this, put the slices in the acidulated water to stop them from discoloring. Drain the Jerusalem artichokes and add them to the pan along with the broth and salt. Bring to a simmer, cover, and cook for 20 minutes or until tender.

While the soup is cooking, make the crumbles. Preheat the broiler and lay the bacon on a rimmed baking sheet. Broil for 9 minutes or until crisp. Remove the bacon and place it on a large plate lined with paper towel, saving the grease for another meal. As the bacon slices cool, they will harden. Crumble with your hands and set aside.

To make the Leafy Swirl, bring a medium pan of water to a boil and have a large bowl of icy water to one side. When the water is boiling, drop in the kale. Turn off the heat and leave the kale in the water for 20 seconds until wilted. Drain and transfer to the cold water to stop the cooking and preserve the color. Once cold, squeeze out the excess water.

Put the kale in a blender or food processor with the parsley, oil, lime juice, salt, and 2 tablespoons (30 ml) water. Blend until smooth. Taste and adjust the seasoning. Transfer to a small bowl and wash your blender.

Remove the soup from the heat and transfer to the blender. Carefully blend in batches until smooth and creamy.

Ladle the soup into bowls and top with the leafy swirl and sprinkling of crumbled bacon.

DIGESTION 101 SALAD
WITH HORSERADISH BEET DRESSING

SERVES 4 AS A SIDE
PREP TIME: 20 MINUTES

SALAD

1 medium endive, base cut off and leaves separated

1 medium fennel bulb, sliced

½ English cucumber, thinly sliced

⅓ bunch watercress, roughly chopped

1 cup (50 g) broccoli sprouts

¼ cup (16 g) chopped fresh dill

½ cup (48 g) fresh mint leaves

1 avocado, sliced

DRESSING
(MAKES ¾ CUP [185 ML])

3 oz (85 g) beet, peeled and chopped

1 teaspoon freshly grated horseradish

½ cup (125 ml) extra virgin olive oil

3 tablespoons (45 ml) raw apple cider vinegar

½ teaspoon raw honey

Pinch Himalayan pink salt

Pinch black pepper

The clue is in the title: Watercress, endive, broccoli sprouts, and apple cider vinegar all support healthy digestion and detoxification. Avocados and olive oil are the healthy fats that stimulate the release of bile. And the star of this salad is the beet, Mother Nature's cleanser. Beets encourage the flow of bile, which aids fat digestion and the removal of toxins through the GI tract. There's more dressing than you need here, so keep the rest in the refrigerator for many more delicious meals.

To make the salad, add the endive, fennel, cucumber, watercress, sprouts, dill, and mint to a large bowl. Mix together well. Add the avocado and gently mix to combine.

To make the dressing, add the beet, horseradish, oil, apple cider vinegar, honey, salt, and pepper to a blender. Blend until smooth, and adjust the oil and seasoning to taste.

Drizzle the dressing over the salad, Jackson Pollock–style, immediately before serving.

Keep unused dressing in a jar and refrigeratefor up to 1 week.

RECIPE IMAGE APPEARS ON PAGE 20.

1

Black pepper	
AIP COMPLIANT	Omit black pepper.
FREEZER-FRIENDLY	No
LOW FODMAP	No
COCONUT-FREE	Yes

SHREDDED BRUSSELS SPROUTS
WITH LEMON & SUMAC

SERVES 4
AS A SIDE

PREP TIME:
10 MINUTES

COOK TIME:
10 MINUTES

2 tablespoons (30 ml)
extra virgin olive oil

1½ lb (675 g) Brussels
sprouts, cut into ⅛-inch
(3-mm) slices

Zest of 1 lemon

1 cup (60 g) chopped fresh
curly parsley

½ teaspoon sumac

Sumac has many health benefits, including helping to regulate blood sugar levels, decreasing cholesterol levels, and acting as a pain reliever. It's also a great spice to use in cooking and works beautifully with Brussels sprouts and lemon. In fact, sumac might just be my new favorite spice.

Heat the oil in a large sauté pan and add the Brussels sprouts. Sauté for 10 to 12 minutes until tender.

Remove from the heat and stir in the lemon zest and parsley. Sprinkle with sumac and serve.

Sumac	1
AIP COMPLIANT Omit sumac.	
FREEZER-FRIENDLY Yes	
LOW FODMAP No	
COCONUT-FREE Yes	

BROTH-BRAISED
PEAS WITH MINT

SERVES 4
AS A SIDE

PREP TIME:
20 MINUTES

COOK TIME:
5 TO 10 MINUTES

1 cup (250 ml) chicken
bone broth

8 asparagus spears,
chopped

1 13 oz (375 g) package
frozen peas

1 tablespoon (15 ml) lemon
juice

Zest of 1 lemon

1 large endive, base cut off
and leaves separated

7 inner leaves of a romaine
lettuce, roughly torn

½ cup (48 g) chopped fresh
mint

Handful pea shoots

Whenever I think of this recipe, I imagine warm, sunny, vitamin D–filled days. It's summer in a bowl the whole year round. This recipe uses frozen peas but do make use of freshly podded whenever you get the chance. If you're still looking for the taste of sunshine and have reintroduced egg yolks, serve the peas with some Mint Mayonnaise (page 81) on the side.

Heat the broth in a large sauté pan and add the asparagus. Bring to a simmer and add the peas and lemon juice.

Bring back to a simmer and cook for a couple of minutes until everything has heated through and the asparagus is tender.

Remove from the heat and stir in the remaining ingredients. Serve immediately.

RECIPE IMAGE APPEARS ON PAGE 44.

1

Peas

AIP COMPLIANT Omit peas and
double up on asparagus.

FREEZER-FRIENDLY Yes

LOW FODMAP No

COCONUT-FREE Yes

ROASTED GREEN BEANS
WITH OLIVE GREMOLATA

SERVES 4
AS A SIDE

PREP TIME:
20 MINUTES

COOK TIME:
15 MINUTES

GREEN BEANS

1 lb (450 g) green
beans, tops trimmed

1 tablespoon (15 ml) extra
virgin olive oil

Flaky sea salt

GREMOLATA

¼ cup (25 g) halved green
olives, finely chopped

¼ cup (25 g) halved black
olives, finely chopped

½ small fennel bulb,
finely chopped

½ cup (30 g) finely chopped
fresh flat-leaf parsley

Zest of ½ large orange

2 tablespoons (30 ml)
orange juice

3 tablespoons (45 ml)
extra virgin olive oil

I love the simplicity of lightly steamed green beans, but roasting and serving with a gremolata does take them a level or two skyward. Heating up the baking sheet beforehand ensures the beans start roasting as soon as they're in the oven, and ultimately spend less time there.

Put a roasting tray in the oven and preheat to 400°F (200°C, or gas mark 6).

To make the green beans, put the beans in a large bowl and pour over the avocado oil. Toss with your hands to coat. Remove the hot roasting tray and add the beans. Sprinkle with sea salt and roast for 12 minutes, or until tender and lightly blistered.

To make the gremolata, combine the olives, fennel, parsley, orange zest and juice, and oil in a medium bowl. Put the beans on a serving platter and spoon the gremolata over the top.

Green beans	1
AIP COMPLIANT Sub broccoli for green beans.	
FREEZER-FRIENDLY Green beans	
LOW FODMAP Yes	
COCONUT-FREE Yes	

CUMIN-ROASTED SALMON
WITH PUMPKIN & ARUGULA

SERVES 4

PREP TIME:
15 MINUTES

COOK TIME:
40 MINUTES

1 teaspoon ground cumin

½ teaspoon ground cinnamon

½ teaspoon ground turmeric

3 tablespoons (45 ml) avocado oil, divided

1 lb (450 g) fillet wild salmon, skin on

1 small pumpkin or winter squash, cut into thick wedges

¾ teaspoon dried thyme

Pinch flaky sea salt

Handful arugula leaves

Extra virgin olive oil

Salmon, like all fish, is easily digested. It also contains more anti-inflammatory omega-3 fatty acids than most others and is high in vitamin D and selenium, deficiencies of which have been linked with autoimmune disease. Choose wild salmon, if possible; nutritionally inferior farmed fish contain antibiotics and other toxins. Cumin's earthy bittersweetness complements the fatty acid–rich salmon and sweet pumpkin really well. It's a lovely combination of flavors.

Preheat the oven to 400°F (200°C, or gas mark 6).

Put the salmon on a rimmed baking sheet. Mix the spices with 1½ tablespoons (23 ml) oil in a small bowl. Brush over the salmon flesh and put in the fridge to marinate while the pumpkin is cooking.

Place the pumpkin in a large roasting pan and drizzle over the remaining oil. Sprinkle with thyme and salt and bake for 30 minutes, turning halfway through the cooking time.

Remove the roasting pan from the oven and push the pumpkin wedges to one side. Place the salmon in the middle and return to the oven. Cook for 8 minutes, or until the salmon is just cooked. Remove from the oven and let the pan sit for a couple of minutes.

Remove the skin from the salmon and flake into large pieces. Arrange on a large serving platter with the pumpkin, and scatter over the arugula.

Drizzle over some extra virgin olive oil and serve.

1

Cumin

AIP COMPLIANT Omit cumin.

FREEZER-FRIENDLY Yes

LOW FODMAP Sub melted coconut oil for avocado oil. Use kabocha squash.

COCONUT-FREE Yes

MUSTARD-BAKED YAM WEDGES
WITH DANDELION-DULSE RELISH

SERVES 4

PREP TIME:
30 MINUTES

COOK TIME:
35 MINUTES

YAM WEDGES

2 tablespoons (18 g)
yellow mustard powder

Pinch fine Himalayan
pink salt

Pinch black pepper
(Stage 1, optional)

2 lb (900 g) yams,
cut into long wedges

3 tablespoons (45 ml)
extra virgin olive oil

RELISH

1 packed cup (about
½ bunch) chopped red
dandelion greens

1 cup (60 g) chopped fresh
curly parsley

2 tablespoons (2.2 g) mixed
sea vegetable flakes,
such as dulse, kelp, nori,
wakame, and sea lettuce

Zest of 1 lemon

2 tablespoons (30 ml)
lemon juice

2 cloves garlic, minced

1 tablespoon (8.6 g)
capers, rinsed well

½ cup (125 ml) extra
virgin olive oil

Mustard gives these baked yams a nice little kick, but you can omit it and this dish will still be delicious. Sea vegetables are super rich in minerals, and dandelion leaves are a potent liver/gallbladder cleanser, so they are extremely beneficial for digestive health. The relish is quite bitter on its own, but it's fantastic paired with the sweetness of yams. The yams are also delicious with the Mint Mayonnaise (page 81), and I love eating the relish with my morning Scromelette (page 90).

Preheat the oven to 400°F (200°C, or gas mark 6). Line two large baking sheets with parchment paper.

To make the yam wedges, combine the mustard powder, salt, and black pepper (if using) in a small bowl. Put the yam wedges in a large bowl, pour over the oil, and, using your hands, toss the wedges until they are well coated. Sprinkle over the mustard mixture and place the wedges onto the baking sheet, leaving space between each one to prevent them from steaming. Bake for 30 to 35 minutes, turning halfway through the cooking time.

Meanwhile, make the relish. Put the dandelion greens, parsley, sea vegetable flakes, lemon zest and juice, garlic, capers, and oil in a food processor. Blitz until combined but still quite chunky. Taste and adjust the flavors as necessary. Transfer to a small bowl.

Places the wedges on a large serving platter with the relish alongside.

RECIPE IMAGE APPEARS
ON PAGE 14.

Mustard	
AIP COMPLIANT Omit mustard and black pepper.	
FREEZER-FRIENDLY Yes	
LOW FODMAP 3 yam wedges. Omit relish.	
COCONUT-FREE Yes	

1

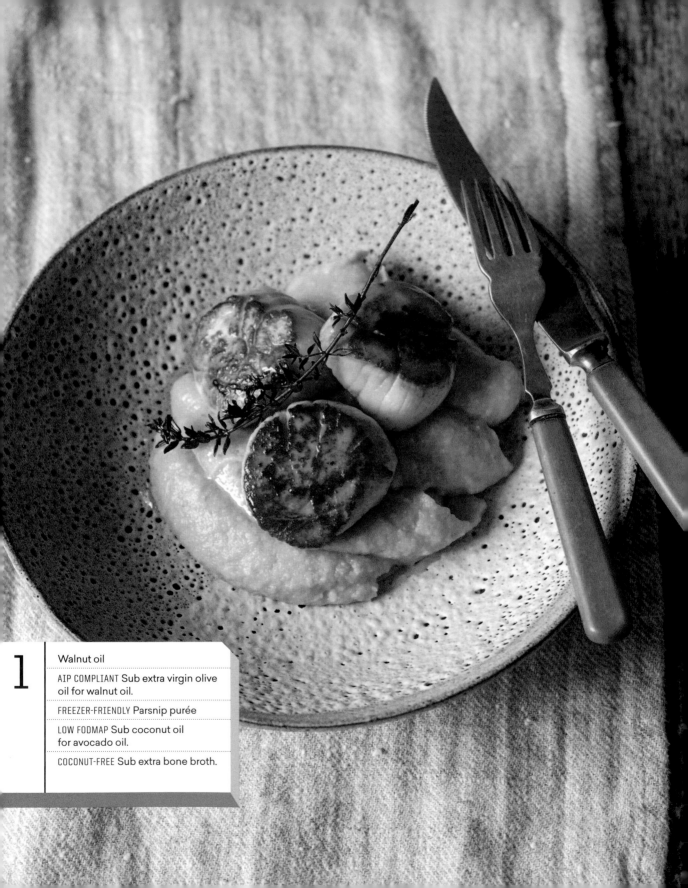

1

Walnut oil

AIP COMPLIANT Sub extra virgin olive oil for walnut oil.

FREEZER-FRIENDLY Parsnip purée

LOW FODMAP Sub coconut oil for avocado oil.

COCONUT-FREE Sub extra bone broth.

PAN-FRIED SCALLOPS
WITH PURÉED PARSNIP & WALNUT OIL

SERVES 4 TO 5

PREP TIME:
20 MINUTES

COOK TIME:
35 MINUTES

PARSNIP PURÉE

3 tablespoons (42 g) softened lard

2¼ lb (1 kg) parsnips, peeled and chopped into ½-inch (1 cm) cubes

1 cup (250 ml) chicken bone broth

½ cup (125 ml) coconut milk

Pinch Himalayan pink salt

SCALLOPS

12–15 large scallops

Pinch sea salt

1 tablespoon (15 ml) extra virgin olive oil

1 tablespoon (42 g) bacon grease, lard, or other solid fat

4–5 sprigs fresh thyme

Walnut oil

Scallops admittedly make a fairly pricey meal, but if you want to treat yourself to a restaurant-quality dinner from the comfort of your dining room, you won't regret it. Try to use bacon grease for this recipe: The combination of scallops, bacon, and parsnips is fantastic.

To make the parsnip purée, heat a sauté pan on medium and add the lard and parsnips. Sauté for 4 to 5 minutes; then stir in the broth, coconut milk, and salt. Cover the pan and continue cooking over low heat for 30 minutes, or until the parsnips are very tender. Put the parsnips in a food processor and slowly add enough of the liquid to make a silky-smooth, mash-like purée. Taste and add more salt if needed. Wipe out the pan with a paper towel.

To make the scallops, pat them dry with paper towels and season with sea salt. Put the sauté pan over high heat, then add the oil, bacon grease, scallops, and thyme. Cook for 2 minutes on each side until just opaque.

Spoon the parsnip purée onto plates and top with the scallops. Pour pan juices over the scallops and add a small drizzle of walnut oil.

CHICKEN WITH LIME GRAVY

SERVES 6 TO 8

PREP TIME: 15 MINUTES

COOK TIME: 50 MINUTES

3 lb (1.4 kg) pasture-raised whole chicken

1 teaspoon ground cumin

1 teaspoon ground coriander

2 teaspoons fenugreek leaves

½ teaspoon ground cinnamon

⅛ teaspoon ground mace

Pinch sea salt

Zest of 2 limes

3 tablespoons (45 ml) avocado oil

¾ cup (185 ml) chicken bone broth

1 tablespoon (15 ml) lime juice

1 teaspoon arrowroot starch

Cutting out the back bone and then flattening is a great way to cook a chicken. It cooks faster than when roasting whole, and you get a raw piece of the carcass for broth making. As you build up the number of fruit- and berry-based spice reintroductions, have fun experimenting with your own blends. Whatever you choose, it will be delicious.

Preheat the oven to 400°F (200°C, or gas mark 6).

Place the chicken on a board, breast side down. With a pair of poultry shears or strong kitchen scissors, cut along either side of the backbone. Remove the bone and keep for making your next batch of broth. Turn the chicken over and push down on the breastbone to flatten the chicken. Place in a small ovenproof pan and tuck the wings behind the neck area.

Mix together the spices, salt, lime zest, and avocado oil in a small bowl.

Using a brush, or the back of a small spoon, cover the chicken skin with the spice paste. Roast in the hot oven for 50 minutes, or until cooked through.

Remove the chicken from the oven and transfer to a large plate. Allow it to rest while you make the gravy.

Scrape the sediment from the bottom of the roasting pan and pour in the broth and lime juice. Bring to a simmer. Mix the arrowroot with 1 tablespoon (15 ml) water in a small bowl and pour into the pan juices. Stir for 2 to 3 minutes until thickened. Press through a sieve into a warm jug and serve.

1

Cumin and coriander

AIP COMPLIANT Omit cumin and coriander.

FREEZER-FRIENDLY Yes

LOW FODMAP Sub extra virgin olive oil for avocado oil.

COCONUT-FREE Yes

NORDIC LAMB GRATIN

SERVES 6

PREP TIME:
25 MINUTES

COOK TIME:
90 MINUTES

1½ lb (675 g) ground lamb

2 tablespoons lard or
other solid fat, divided

1 large red onion,
chopped

3 oz (85 g) shiitake
mushrooms, sliced

2 teaspoons dried juniper
berries, lightly crushed

2 large cloves garlic,
minced

1 tablespoon chopped
fresh rosemary

1 tablespoon fresh thyme

1¾ cups (435 ml)
chicken bone broth

Pinch sea salt

1 cup fresh or frozen
cranberries

½ cup coconut cream
(see note)

2 tablespoons chopped
fresh dill

1½ lb (675 g) celeriac
(celery root)

12 oz (340 g) white
sweet potato, peeled

Lamb has a richer flavor than beef that I really enjoy, and, because it contains more fat than other red meats, it's less likely to dry out. It's also worth knowing that the majority of sheep are grass-fed so it's a good option if the price of grass-fed beef is overstretching your budget. If you don't care for lamb, use beef or bison instead. Juniper berries, which are commonly used in Scandinavia, are known for their anti-inflammatory and antioxidant properties.

Heat a large sauté pan or frying pan on medium-high and cook the lamb for 5 minutes. You shouldn't need any fat as lamb is a fatty meat. Set a colander over a bowl and strain the lamb.

Put 1 tablespoon of the solid fat in the pan and sauté the onions on medium-low for 4 minutes. Add the shiitakes and juniper berries, and cook for 4 to 5 minutes until softened. Stir in the garlic, rosemary, and thyme, and cook for 1 to 2 minutes. Stir in the lamb, broth, and salt, and cover the pan. Simmer for 30 minutes until the juices are almost absorbed. Add the cranberries and coconut cream. Cook gently for 15 minutes until the sauce is rich and creamy. Stir in the dill. Taste and adjust the seasoning if needed.

Meanwhile, preheat the oven to 400°F (200°C, or gas mark 6).

Slice the celeriac and sweet potato into ⅛-inch (3 mm) rounds, keeping them separate. Steam the slices for 5 minutes, or until just tender.

Melt the remaining tablespoon of solid fat in a small pan. Transfer the meat sauce to a 2½-pint (50 fl oz) baking dish and add the vegetable slices in alternate concentric circles, overlapping and layering until you have used them all. You should have about three layers, depending on your dish. Brush the top layer with the fat to encourage it to brown. Sprinkle sea salt over the top.

Place the dish on a baking sheet and cook for 30 minutes. Turn the heat up to 425°F (220°C, or gas mark 7) for the final 10 minutes. Remove from the oven and serve.

NOTE **Refrigerate a can (400 ml) of coconut milk the night before you make the recipe. Turn the can upside down, open with a can opener and pour off the water. The cream is left behind.**

Juniper berries

AIP COMPLIANT Omit juniper.

FREEZER-FRIENDLY Yes

LOW FODMAP Sub green part of leek for onion. Omit mushrooms. Omit garlic.

COCONUT-FREE Sub extra broth.

1

SLOW-ROASTED PORK BELLY
WITH STAR ANISE & FENNEL

SERVES 6

PREP TIME:
20 MINUTES,
PLUS OPTIONAL
CHILLING TIME

COOK TIME: 4 HOURS

2 large whole star anise

2 tablespoons (11.6 g)
fennel seeds

2 tablespoons flaky sea
salt

4 lb (2 kg) pork belly,
scored

2 tablespoons (30 ml)
avocado or coconut oil

3 onions, quartered

1 large fennel bulb,
quartered

1 cup (250 ml) hot chicken
bone broth

If you ask your butcher to score the meat for you, this recipe can be prepped in minutes. If you have the time, prepare the pork belly in advance: Press the seed rub into the skin and refrigerate, uncovered, the night before you want to eat. Doing so will dry out the skin and you'll have the crispiest crackling imaginable. A family favorite!

Bring the pork to room temperature for at least an hour before cooking. Preheat the oven to 475°F (240°C, or gas mark 9).

Pound the star anise, fennel seeds, and salt with a pestle and mortar and rub into the pork fat, making sure the spices go down into the crevices. Drizzle over the oil, rubbing it over the fat and brushing off the excess.

Arrange the onions and fennel like a trivet in a large roasting pan and place the pork over the top. Roast for 45 minutes.

Reduce the oven temperature to 300°F (150°C, or gas mark 2) and continue cooking for 3 hours until you can easily pull the meat apart. Transfer the pork to a board or warm serving dish and set aside while you make the gravy.

Remove the onions and fennel and put in a blender with the broth. Blend until smooth, adding more hot broth if needed. Reheat and strain into a jug.

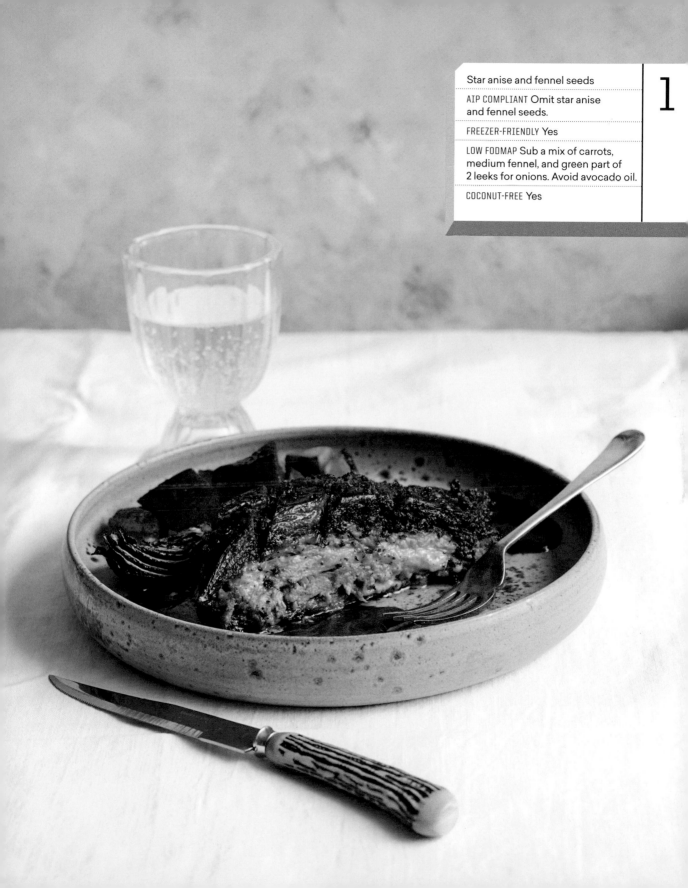

Star anise and fennel seeds

AIP COMPLIANT Omit star anise and fennel seeds.

FREEZER-FRIENDLY Yes

LOW FODMAP Sub a mix of carrots, medium fennel, and green part of 2 leeks for onions. Avoid avocado oil.

COCONUT-FREE Yes

1

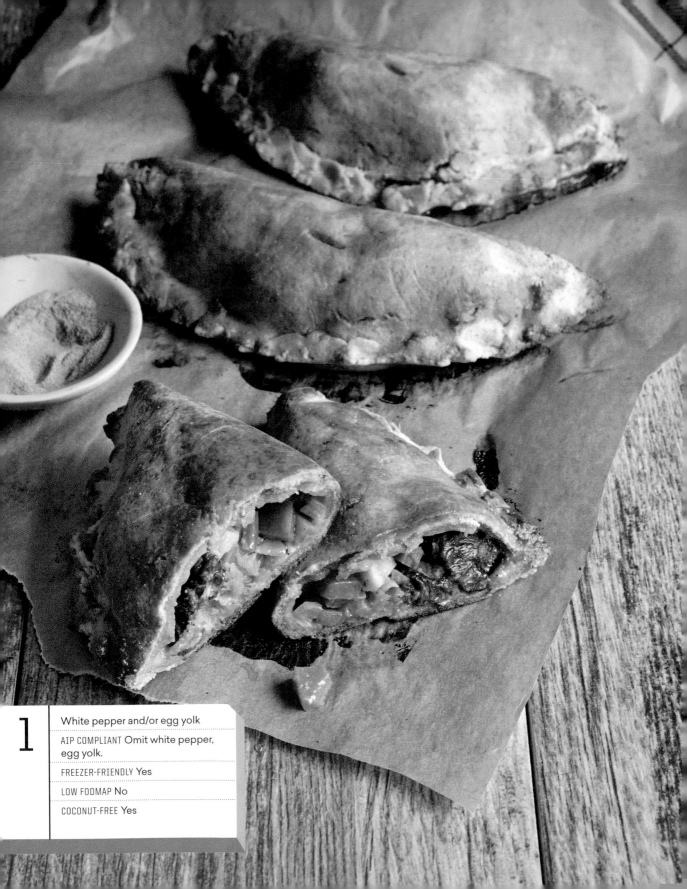

1

White pepper and/or egg yolk

AIP COMPLIANT Omit white pepper, egg yolk.

FREEZER-FRIENDLY Yes

LOW FODMAP No

COCONUT-FREE Yes

TRADITIONAL-ISH
CORNISH PASTY

MAKES 4

PREP TIME:
70 MINUTES (INCLUDING
RESTING PASTRY)

COOK TIME:
45 MINUTES

I spent the majority of my childhood in Cornwall; my parents still live there today. I grew up eating home-cooked meals, and it was always a treat to have a pasty—on those rare occasions when my mum didn't want to cook or we nagged until she gave in. So, believe me when I say this recipe is as near to a Cornish pasty as you're going to get with AIP ingredients. It is so good!

PASTRY

1 cup (153 g) cassava flour

⅓ cup (44 g) tapioca flour

1 teaspoon gelatin

1 cup (225 g) cold cooked
mashed white sweet
potato

Pinch sea salt

⅓ cup (80 ml) avocado oil

⅓ cup (80 ml) room
temperature water plus
4 tablespoons (60 ml)

Beaten egg yolk or coconut
milk for brushing

FILLING

7 oz (200 g) rutabaga,
peeled and cut into
¼-inch (6 mm) cubes

4 oz (110 g) white sweet
potato, peeled and cut into
¼-inch (6 mm) cubes

1 small yellow onion,
finely chopped

½ lb (225 g) beef skirt
steak, cut into ¼-inch
(6 mm) cubes

Pinch sea salt

Pinch white pepper

To make the pastry, put the flours, gelatin, sweet potato, and salt in a large bowl and, using a couple of knives and a criss-cross action, cut in the sweet potato as though it were butter. Alternatively, use a pastry blender. Once the sweet potato resembles small chunks of butter, put the avocado oil in a jug with ⅓ cup (80 ml) water and mix together. Using just one knife now, mix as you slowly pour in the oil and water mixture. Add extra water by the teaspoon until the mixture starts to come together. Switch to using one hand, and bring together to form a firm dough.

Divide into 4 pieces and shape into 1-inch (2.5 cm) discs. Cover with plastic wrap and refrigerate for 30 minutes.

When you are ready to cook your pasties, preheat the oven to 350°F (175°C, or gas mark 4). Line a large rimmed baking sheet with parchment paper.

Roll the pastry between two pieces of parchment until it's a circle ¼-inch (6 mm) thick and roughly 7 inches (18 cm) in diameter.

To make the filling, divide the rutabaga, sweet potato, and onion between the pastry rounds and arrange in a mound along the middle. Place the beef over the top of the vegetables, followed by a sprinkling of salt and white pepper.

With hands either side of the parchment paper, bring the pastry to join the other side in a semicircle and crimp the edges. Place the pasty onto the lined baking sheet, with the crimped side down against the parchment paper. Use a knife to make a slit in the top of the pasty to allow steam to escape. Glaze the top with egg yolk if you have reintroduced it, or else a little coconut milk. Repeat with the other three pasties.

Bake for 40 to 45 minutes until golden. Stand for 5 to 10 minutes before eating and be mindful that the inside will be piping hot.

NY STEAK
WITH CAULIFLOWER, CAPERS & MUSTARD CRUMBS

SERVES 2 TO 3

PREP TIME:
15 MINUTES

COOK TIME:
15 MINUTES

STEAK

1 teaspoon (5 ml)
extra virgin olive oil

Pinch sea salt

2 (6 oz [170 g]) New York
striploin steaks

CRUMBS

2 teaspoons (10 ml)
extra virgin olive oil

1¼ cups riced cauliflower

1 large garlic clove,
finely chopped

1 teaspoon Windfall
Country Mustard (page 79)

1 tablespoon (8.6 g)
capers, rinsed and roughly
chopped

2 tablespoons (4 g)
roughly chopped fresh
flat-leaf parsley

This recipe couldn't be any simpler, and yet it looks—and tastes— good enough to be on a restaurant menu. Have everything on hand before you start, because it's unbelievably quick. The secret is to get a really good- quality piece of meat and, once cooked, allow it to rest before slicing.

To make the steak, place a heavy-based frying pan over medium-high heat. Sprinkle a little salt onto both sides of the steaks. Using a pair of tongs, hold the steaks upright on the hot pan for 1 to 2 minutes, fat side down along the edge. This allows the fat to render into the pan. Next, lay the steaks down and cook for 3 minutes on the first side. Turn them over and cook for 1 minute for a rare steak. This timing obviously depends on the thickness of your steak.

If your steak doesn't have any fat along the side, put a teaspoon of oil on a large plate, coat the steaks in the oil and then sprinkle both sides with a little salt. Heat your frying pan over medium-high heat and add the steak. Cook on the first side for 3 minutes, then turn over and continue for 2 minutes for a rare steak, or longer if you prefer it cooked more. As with the first method, the exact timing will depend on how thick your steak is.

Transfer to a warm plate and allow to rest. Do not wipe out the pan.

To make the crumbs, turn the heat down to medium. Put 2 teaspoons (10 ml) of oil in the pan and add the riced cauliflower. Spread it out so it doesn't steam; cook the cauliflower as though you are toasting breadcrumbs. Sauté the cauliflower rice for 2 to 3 minutes, until just tender and pale brown (it will already have taken on some color from the steak). Add the remaining ingredients and continue cooking for 1 minute.

Slice the steak into thin strips and lay out on plates. Top with the mustard crumbs and serve immediately.

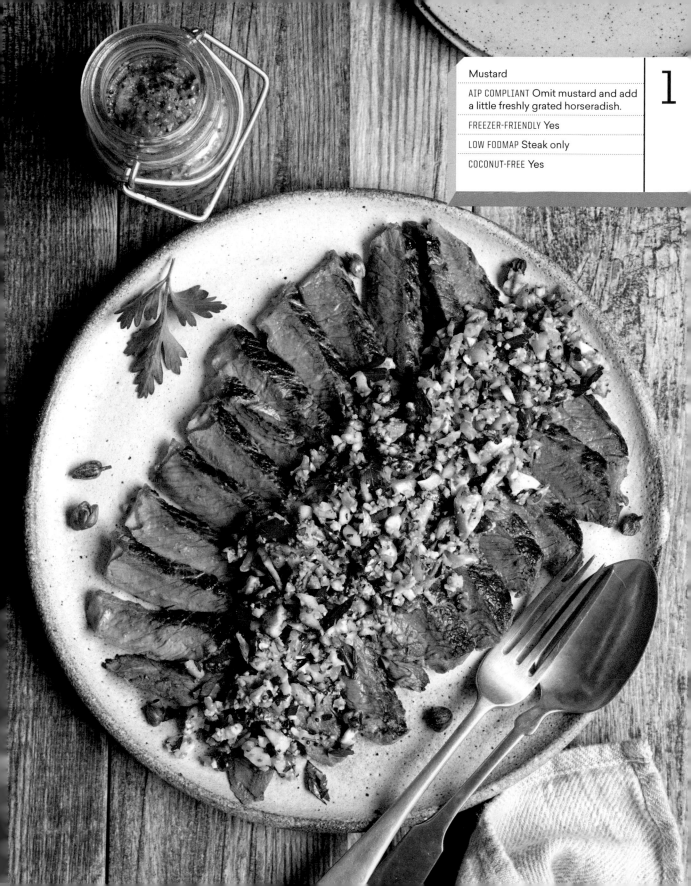

Mustard

AIP COMPLIANT Omit mustard and add a little freshly grated horseradish.

FREEZER-FRIENDLY Yes

LOW FODMAP Steak only

COCONUT-FREE Yes

1

PEAR, RASPBERRY & CARDAMOM
GALETTE

SERVES 8

PREP TIME:
40 MINUTES, PLUS
CHILLING TIME

COOK TIME:
40 MINUTES

PASTRY

1 cup (153 g) cassava flour

¾ cup (85 g) tigernut flour

1 tablespoon (8.25 g)
arrowroot

Pinch sea salt

4 oz (110 g) cold lard, cut
into small cubes

1 tablespoon (9 g) coconut
sugar

¼ cup (61.3 g) pumpkin
purée

¼ cup (60 ml) plus 3
tablespoons (45 ml)
ice-cold water

FILLING

1½ teaspoons coconut
sugar

½ teaspoon ground
cardamom

4 ripe pears, peeled,
quartered, and thinly sliced

½ cup (65 g) fresh
raspberries

2 teaspoons (10 ml)
melted coconut oil

I like to use my food processor to bring this pastry together. It's quite forgiving, so if you have any cracks or gaps, take a bit of pastry from an outer edge and patch it up where necessary. It's meant to look rustic, after all. Pear, raspberry, and cardamom make a delightful combination, or you can fill the pastry with anything you like: Apple and cinnamon, peach and vanilla, or banana and cardamom all spring to mind.

To make the pastry, put the flours, arrowroot, and salt in the bowl of your food processor and pulse a couple of times to combine. Add the lard and pulse again until the mixture resembles coarse breadcrumbs. Next, add the coconut sugar and pulse once or twice more.

Mix the pumpkin purée with ¼ cup (60 ml) cold water and, with the motor running, slowly add to the flour mixture. Trickle in extra cold water until the mixture just begins to hold together; stop pulsing. You may not need all the water, or you may need more. Sprinkle a little cassava flour on your work top and tip out the pastry mix. Bring the mixture to form a dough and flatten into a thick disc. Cover with plastic wrap and chill in the refrigerator for at least 30 minutes.

Cut two pieces of parchment paper a little larger than the size of your baking sheet and place the pastry dough between the two. Flatten with your hands and then roll out the dough with a rolling pin, until it's roughly ⅛ inch (3 mm) thick and 12½ (31 cm) inches in diameter.

Put the baking sheet in the oven and preheat to 400°F (200°C, or gas mark 6).

To make the filling, mix the coconut sugar and cardamom in a small bowl.

Leaving a 2-inch (5 cm) border from the edge of the pastry, sprinkle over half the cardamom sugar over the dough. Arrange the pear slices so they are over-lapping one another and scatter the raspberries over the top.

Pull up the parchment on all sides to guide the edges of the pastry back onto the fruit, overlapping and pressing down lightly as you go around the galette, leaving the fruits exposed.

Lightly brush the pastry and fruits with the melted coconut oil and sprinkle over the remaining cardamom sugar.

Bake for 40 minutes, or until the pastry is just firm. This is best eaten warm on the day of making.

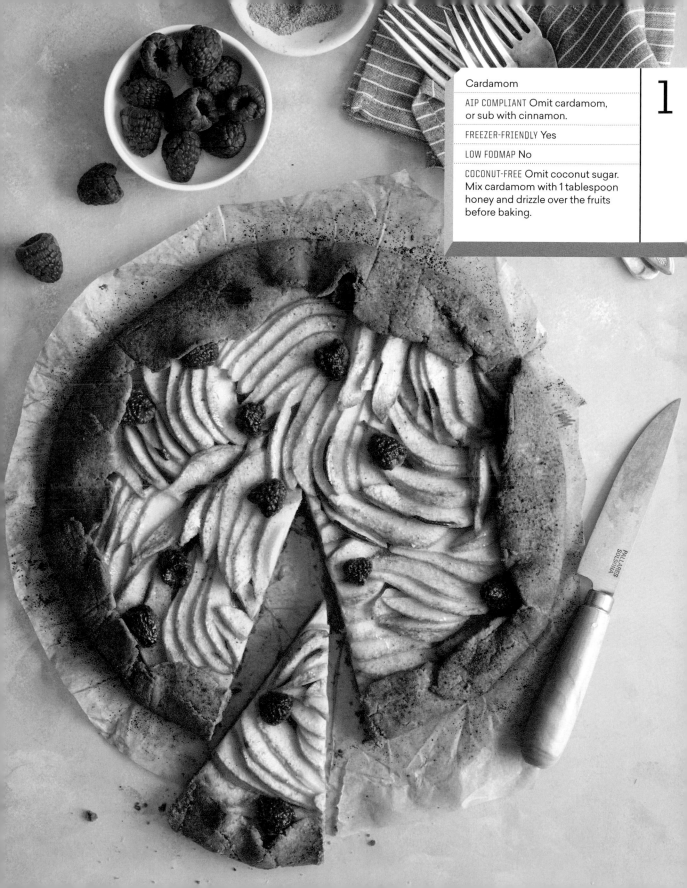

Cardamom

AIP COMPLIANT Omit cardamom, or sub with cinnamon.

FREEZER-FRIENDLY Yes

LOW FODMAP No

COCONUT-FREE Omit coconut sugar. Mix cardamom with 1 tablespoon honey and drizzle over the fruits before baking.

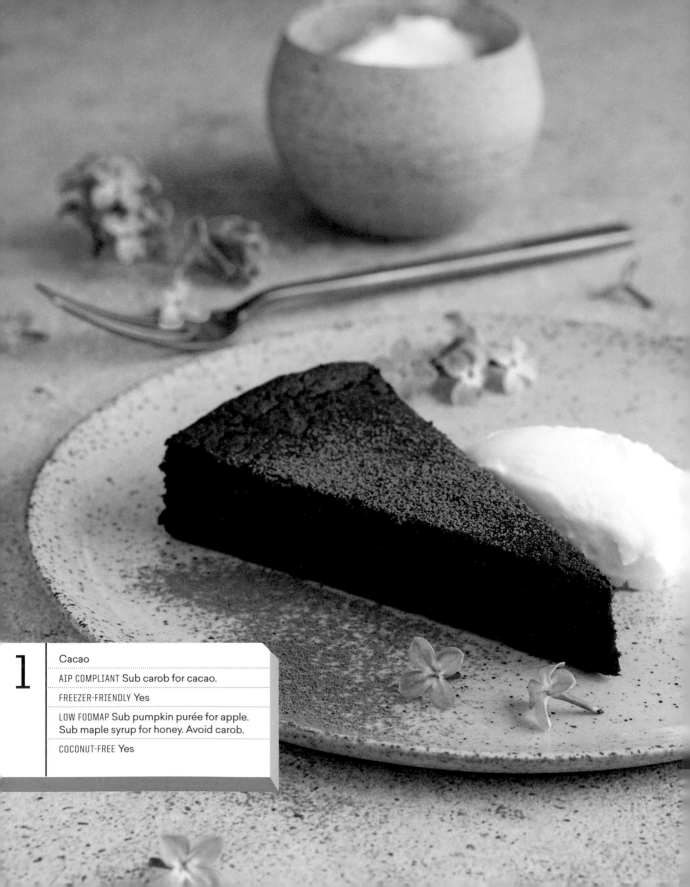

1

Cacao

AIP COMPLIANT Sub carob for cacao.

FREEZER-FRIENDLY Yes

LOW FODMAP Sub pumpkin purée for apple.
Sub maple syrup for honey. Avoid carob.

COCONUT-FREE Yes

CHOCOLATE SWEET POTATO
MUD CAKE

SERVES 8

PREP TIME:
45 MINUTES

COOK TIME:
90 MINUTES

1 lb (450 g) white sweet
potato, peeled and
chopped

1 medium sweet red apple,
peeled, cored, and chopped

½ cup (100 g) softened lard

2 tablespoons (30 ml)
honey

Pinch sea salt

¾ cup (85 g) tigernut flour

¼ cup (21.5 g) raw cacao
powder

1 teaspoon ground
cinnamon

½ teaspoon baking soda

GELATIN EGG

1 tablespoon (10 g)
grass-fed gelatin

½ teaspoon raw apple
cider vinegar

2 tablespoons (30 ml)
hot water

This more-ish cake gets most of its sweetness from sweet potatoes and apple. It includes a small amount of honey to take the bitterness off the cacao. If you enjoy bitter chocolate, leave the honey out, and definitely omit it if using carob, as it is naturally sweet. This cake has a melt-in-the-mouth moist, fudgey texture. It is delicious on its own, or serve it with a light dusting of raw cacao powder and a spoonful of coconut yogurt. Totally addictive—just don't forget the rest of your veggies need to come from elsewhere!

Steam the sweet potatoes for 15 to 20 minutes until soft. Meanwhile, put the apple in a small pan with 2 tablespoons (30 ml) water. Bring to a simmer, cover, and cook for 15 minutes or until soft. Put the sweet potatoes and apple onto separate plates and mash well with a fork while still hot. Cool completely. You should have 1½ cups of sweet potato purée and ½ cup of apple purée.

Put a baking sheet in the oven and preheat to 325°F (170°C, or gas mark 3). Line an 8-inch (20 cm) cake tin with parchment paper. Cross a couple of long strips of parchment underneath the lining, letting them hang over the edges of the tin so you can lift the cake out, rather than turn the tin upside down. Alternatively use a parchment-lined springform tin.

Put the apple purée, lard, honey, and salt in the bowl of a stand mixer, or use a hand mixer, and combine until fluffy. Add the tigernut flour, cacao powder, cinnamon, and baking soda and mix again. Scrape down the sides of the bowl. Put the sweet potato mash in the bowl and switch the motor back on low.

Make the gelatin egg. Put the gelatin in a small bowl; put the apple cider vinegar and water in a separate small bowl. Pour the liquid onto the gelatin and whisk until frothy. Tip into the cake mixture, increase the motor speed, and blend for 5 to 6 seconds until thoroughly combined.

Spoon the mixture into the cake tin and level the top. Cook for 1 hour, or until firm on the top and coming away from the sides of the parchment. Leave in the tin for 45 minutes before carefully turning out onto a plate.

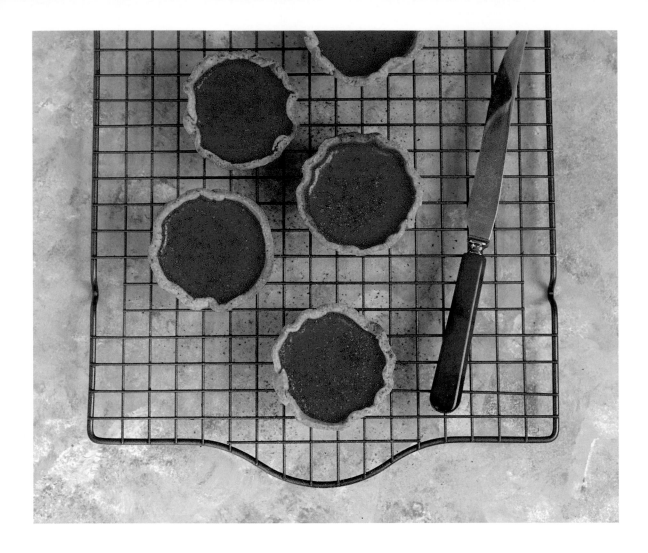

MINI
CUSTARD TARTS

MAKES 6

PREP TIME:
45 MINUTES, PLUS
CHILLING TIME

COOK TIME:
35 MINUTES

These little tarts are rich and utterly delicious. The secret to successful pastry is handling it as little as possible, so I've left these tart shells in a rustic shape, pushing them only very lightly into the muffin tin. This also makes them easy to remove once baked. If you freeze the leftover egg whites in batches of three, you'll be able to make two batches of the Maple Meringues on page 116 once you've introduced them.

PASTRY

½ cup (76 g) cassava flour

¼ cup (35 g) coconut flour

Pinch sea salt

1½ oz (45 g) cold lard, cut into small cubes

1½ teaspoons coconut sugar

1 egg yolk

⅓ cup (80 ml) plus 1 tablespoon (15 ml) ice-cold water

CUSTARD

½ cup (125 ml) coconut milk

½ cup (125 ml) coconut cream

5 egg yolks

2 tablespoons (30 ml) honey

Freshly grated nutmeg (optional)

To make the pastry, put the flours and salt in a large bowl and, using a couple of knives and a criss-cross action, cut in the lard until the mixture resembles breadcrumbs. Alternatively, use a pastry blender. Stir in the coconut sugar.

Mix the egg yolk with 3 tablespoons (45 ml) of the cold water and add to the mixture. Mix with just one knife, adding 1 tablespoon (15 ml) of water at a time, until everything has come together. You may not need all the water. Using one hand now, form a dough with the mixture. Flatten into a thick round, cover with plastic wrap, and chill in the refrigerator for at least 30 minutes.

Preheat the oven to 375°F (190°C, or gas mark 5).

Put the pasty between two sheets of parchment paper and roll out to an 11-inch (28 cm) circle. Using a 4-inch (10 cm) cookie cutter, cut out six circles ⅛ inch (3 mm) thick. Gently press each one into the holes of a muffin tin, leaving the top of the pastry flush with the top of the muffin tin. They will be hanging in suspension but don't worry about that. Place in the fridge for 20 to 30 minutes to firm up.

After removing the tin from the fridge, cut out six 4-inch (10 cm) circles from the parchment paper and use them to line the pastry cases. Fill with baking beans or rice and bake for 14 to 15 minutes until the pastry is cooked. Remove from the oven and lift out the parchment circles. Reduce the temperature to 275°F (140°C, or gas mark 1).

To make the custard, put the coconut milk and cream in a medium pan and bring to a simmer. Put the egg yolks and honey in a medium bowl and whisk until pale and fluffy. Pour the hot liquid over the egg mixture, whisking continuously. Strain into a jug.

Pour the custard into the pastry cases, filling up to the top. Grate a little nutmeg over (if using), and return to the oven, being careful not to spill the liquid over the pastry as they may be difficult to remove later. Gently close the oven door and cook for 15 to 16 minutes, or until the tarts are almost set and still wobble slightly in the middle when you gently shake the tin.

Remove from the oven and allow to cool for 30 minutes. Carefully remove the tarts and place them on a wire rack to cool completely. Just before serving, dust with a little more grated nutmeg (if using).

Egg yolk plus nutmeg (optional)	1
AIP COMPLIANT Use the pastry on page 68 and fill with AIP panna cotta (page 158).	
FREEZER-FRIENDLY Pastry	
LOW FODMAP No	
COCONUT-FREE No	

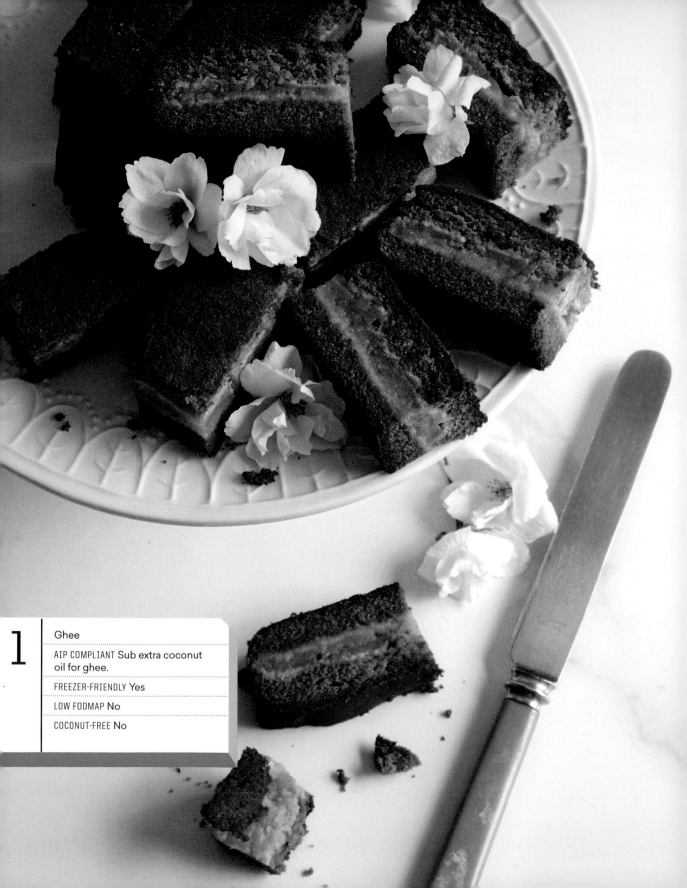

1

Ghee

AIP COMPLIANT Sub extra coconut oil for ghee.

FREEZER-FRIENDLY Yes

LOW FODMAP No

COCONUT-FREE No

TRIPLE APPLE
PIE BARS

MAKES ONE 7-INCH
(18 CM) SQUARE CAKE
PREP TIME: 35 MINUTES
COOK TIME: 45 MINUTES

1 lb (450 g) Pink Lady
apples, peeled, cored,
and chopped

¾ lb (340 g) Braeburn
apples, peeled, cored,
and chopped

6 whole cloves

½ cup (200 g) softened
lard or (109 g) coconut oil

¼ cup (56 g) ghee

¼ cup (85 g) honey

1 cup (140 g) coconut flour

¼ cup (33 g) arrowroot
starch

1 teaspoon baking soda

Pinch sea salt

½ cup (125 ml) coconut
milk

8 oz (225 g) Granny
Smith apple, peeled, cored,
and thinly sliced

GELATIN EGGS

2 tablespoons (20 g)
grass-fed gelatin

1 teaspoon (5 ml) raw
apple cider vinegar

3 tablespoons (45 ml) hot
water from the kettle

I love using different apple varieties together to achieve a balance of sweetness, acidity, and structure. When you combine apples that make the perfect sauce with those that are known to hold up well during baking, the end result is much more interesting. My favorites for purée include Pink Lady, Gala, and Braeburn, but I've also used Fuji and Ambrosia. I'm far more particular about using a Granny Smith for the slices, because it keeps its shape so well and has an acidity that is wonderful against the sweetness of the cake. For more apple combinations in Stage 2, try the Apple & Walnut Crumble recipe (page 117).

Boil a kettle full of water while you prepare your ingredients.

Put the Pink Lady and Braeburn apples in a small pan together with the cloves and ¼ cup (60 ml) water. Cover and cook for 10 to 12 minutes until soft. Remove from the heat, discard the cloves, and mash thoroughly. You should have 1¼ cups (305 g) of purée. Transfer to a plate and cool.

Place a baking sheet in the oven and preheat to 350°F (175°C, or gas mark 4). Line a 7-inch (18 cm) square baking pan with parchment paper.

Put ½ cup (125 g) of the apple purée in the bowl of a stand mixer. Add the lard, ghee, and honey and combine until fluffy. Sift in the coconut flour, arrowroot, baking soda, and salt, and combine.

To make the gelatin eggs, put the gelatin in a small bowl and the apple cider vinegar and water in a separate small bowl. Pour the liquid onto the gelatin, whisk until frothy, and tip into the mixture in the stand mixer. Add the coconut milk, and blend for 4 to 5 seconds until thoroughly combined.

Spoon half the mixture into the prepared tin and level the surface. Spread the remaining apple purée evenly over the mixture and layer the apples slices over the purée. Dot the remaining cake mixture over the top and level the surface again, using your fingers if necessary.

Put the pan onto the hot baking sheet and bake for 40 minutes, or until golden brown, firm to the touch, and coming away from the parchment. Allow to cool in the tin before transferring to a wire rack. The cake will firm up more as it cools. Cut into bars or squares and store in an airtight container.

COFFEE BERRY
COMPOTE

SERVES 4 TO 6

PREP TIME:
10 MINUTES

COOK TIME:
35 MINUTES

6 oz (1¼ cup) blackberries

6 oz (1¼ cup) blueberries

1 teaspoon ground cinnamon

½ cup (125 ml) strong black coffee, cooled

2 tablespoons (30 ml) maple syrup

2 red pears, cored and chopped into ¾-inch (2 cm) chunks

Coffee is avoided in the elimination phase because it's a seed. However, it is known to protect the heart, support cognitive function, and reduce the risk of diabetes, so we introduce it in Stage 1 for occasional use and Stage 2 for regular use. I love a subtle hint of coffee paired with berries, but if you're passionate about your coffee, you can make yours stronger if you like. Both coffee and berries are high in antioxidants so this is a nutritional double whammy.

Preheat the oven to 375°F (190°C, or gas mark 5). Put the fruits in a medium roasting pan.

Put the cinnamon, coffee, and maple syrup in a jug and combine. Pour over the fruits and bake for about 35 minutes, until the pears have softened and the juice is almost syrupy. It becomes more syrupy when cooling.

Spoon into a jar when cool. Eat on its own, or serve with the Buckwheat Tigernut Pancakes (or AIP version) on page 166, the Maple Turmeric Oats on page 170, or coconut yogurt.

1

Coffee (occasional basis)

AIP COMPLIANT Omit coffee.

FREEZER-FRIENDLY Yes

LOW FODMAP Omit pears and blackberries. Add other berries and reduce cooking time to 20 minutes.

COCONUT-FREE Yes

BEET KVASS
WITH ORANGE PEEL & FENNEL

MAKES ONE 3-PINT
(1.5-LITER) JAR

PREP TIME:
20 MINUTES

FERMENTING TIME:
5 TO 7 DAYS

3 medium organic beets,
trimmed and gently
scrubbed

Peel of 1 large orange,
removed with a vegetable
peeler

1 tablespoon (5.8 g) fennel
seeds

1 tablespoon coarse
sea salt

This tangy probiotic drink makes a nice change from kombucha. It also has the added benefit of being a fine liver/gallbladder tonic and digestive aid. Start slowly and build up to around half a cup twice daily, and do purchase organic beets as conventionally grown beets are usually from genetically modified crops.

You will need a 3-pint (1.5 liter) sterilized jar with a tight-fitting lid.

Chop the beets into approximate 1-inch (2.5 cm) pieces and put them in the jar. Add the orange peel, fennel seeds, and salt.

Top up with 5 cups of filtered water, leaving 1 inch (2.5 cm) of space at the top. Put the lid on and give it a shake to dissolve the salt.

Place on your counter for 4 to 7 days until it tastes tangy, "burping" the jar once a day to let any excess buildup of gases escape. The exact fermentation time will depend on your room temperature.

Decant into sterilized bottles if you like, or leave in the jar. Transfer to the refrigerator.

When the kvass is down to the last ¼ cup (60 ml), either top up with water and ferment once again, or use as a starter for a new batch and add the pickled beets to your salads.

RECIPE IMAGE APPEARS ON PAGE 40.

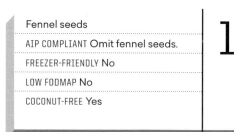

Fennel seeds

AIP COMPLIANT Omit fennel seeds.

FREEZER-FRIENDLY No

LOW FODMAP No

COCONUT-FREE Yes

1

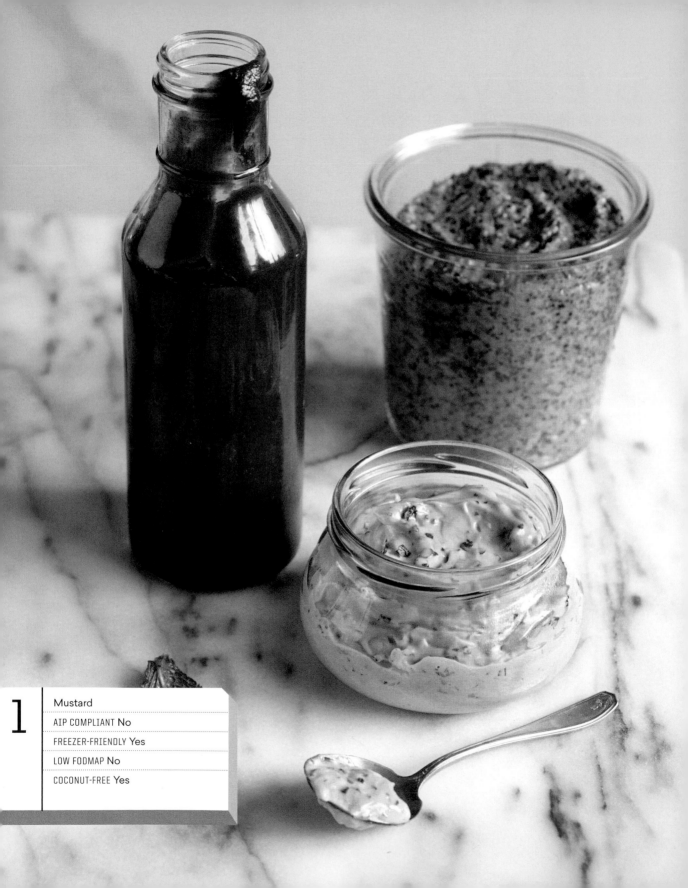

1	Mustard
	AIP COMPLIANT No
	FREEZER-FRIENDLY Yes
	LOW FODMAP No
	COCONUT-FREE Yes

WINDFALL COUNTRY
MUSTARD

MAKES 1¼ CUPS (220 G)

PREP TIME:
20 MINUTES, PLUS
OVERNIGHT SOAKING

COOK TIME:
15 MINUTES

½ cup (88 g) yellow
mustard seeds

½ cup (88 g) brown
mustard seeds

1¼ cup (310 ml) water

½ cup (125 ml) raw apple
cider vinegar

1 red apple, peeled,
cored, and chopped

1 red pear, peeled,
cored, and chopped

1 teaspoon sea salt

Most store-bought mustards contain sugar and other additives, but luckily you can make your own very quickly, and you get to control the ingredients you use. I used a Pink Lady apple and red d'Anjou pear for my mustard, but you can use whatever's available in the grocery store—or whatever fell down in the wind!

You will need a ½ liter capacity sterilized jar.

Put the mustard seeds in a small bowl with the water and apple cider vinegar. Cover and leave to stand overnight.

Put the apple and pear in a small pan, together with 2 tablespoons (30 ml) water. Cook gently for 12 minutes, or until softened. Remove from the heat and purée. Allow to cool.

Put all the ingredients in a blender and blitz well until you have the texture you like. Note, the more you blend, the stronger the mustard will become.

Spoon into a sterilized jar and keep for up to 2 months in the refrigerator.

NIGHTSHADE-FREE
BROWN SAUCE

MAKES 4½ CUPS (FILLS TWO
250 ML PRESERVING JARS,
OR EQUIVALENT)

PREP TIME: 20 MINUTES

COOK TIME: 45 MINUTES

3 (1½ lb or 675 g) Granny
Smith apples, peeled, cored, and
chopped

1 medium red onion, chopped

2 large cloves garlic, minced

1 tablespoon (40 g) tamarind
paste

2 tablespoons (40 g) blackstrap
molasses

10 medjool dates, pitted and
chopped

1½ cups (375 ml) raw apple cider
vinegar

⅓ cup (80 ml) fresh orange juice
(navel, if possible)

½ teaspoon ground cinnamon

½ teaspoon ground allspice

Pinch sea salt

Pinch black pepper

A fruity, tangy sauce that's reminiscent of the one that graces many British tables when chips are on the menu. A little goes a long way. You'll find this is an ideal accompaniment to steak, burgers, fries, tacos, and stews, or for livening up any meal, for that matter. My life is complete now!

Put the apples, onion, garlic, tamarind paste, molasses, dates, apple cider vinegar, orange juice, cinnamon, allspice, salt, and pepper in a large pan. Bring to a boil; then turn down to a simmer and cover. Cook for 45 minutes until everything has broken down and the liquid has almost evaporated.

Transfer the mixture to a blender and blend to a smooth sauce.

Pour into sterilized bottles or jars. Cool and keep in the fridge for one month. Alternatively freeze for up to 3 months.

1

Allspice and black pepper

AIP COMPLIANT Omit allspice and
black pepper.

FREEZER-FRIENDLY Yes

LOW FODMAP No

COCONUT-FREE Yes

MINT
MAYONNAISE

MAKES 1¼ CUPS (400 G)

PREP TIME:
15 MINUTES

3 egg yolks

¼ pint (150 ml) extra
virgin olive oil

¼ pint (150 ml)
avocado oil

Zest of 1 lemon

4 tablespoons (60 ml)
lemon juice

½ cup (48 g) finely chopped
fresh mint

Pinch sea salt

Homemade mayonnaise has so much more flavor than store-bought, and it's simple to make if you take it slowly. Don't throw out your egg whites—you have just the right amount to make the Maple Meringues (page 116). If you're not ready to reintroduce egg whites yet, don't worry: Freeze them individually in small ice cube trays, so you can keep track of how many you have when the time comes. If you'd like an AIP-compliant mayo, see the additional recipe at the bottom.

Put the egg yolks in the small bowl of a food processor and start the motor running. Mix the oils together in a jug and add to the bowl in a slow, steady drizzle. If you add it too quickly the mixture will curdle. Once you have used half of the oil, you can pour the remainder a little more quickly.

If the mixture curdles, it can be rescued. Simply transfer the mixture into a jug and place another egg yolk in the food processor bowl. With the motor running, add the curdled mixture a spoonful at a time.

Once all the oil is incorporated, add the lemon zest and juice, mint, and salt to taste.

For a fully AIP compliant version, blend ½ cup (110 g) coconut cream, ¼ cup (150 ml) mild extra virgin olive oil, pinch of sea salt, zest of 1 lemon, 2 teaspoons (10 ml) lemon juice, and ½ cup (48 g) finely chopped mint leaves. For the coconut cream, refrigerate a can of coconut milk overnight and scoop off the cream that has risen to the top.

Egg yolks	1
AIP COMPLIANT No. See above.	
FREEZER-FRIENDLY No	
LOW FODMAP Sub avocado oil for a light olive oil.	
COCONUT-FREE Yes	

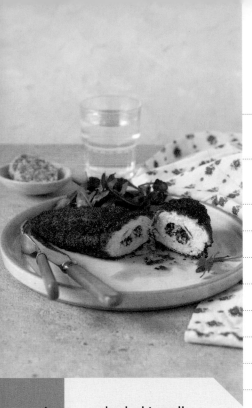

STAGE 2 RECIPES

RECIPE APPEARS ON PAGE 105.

reintroduction foods covered in this chapter

- alcohol (small quantities)
- almonds
- butter
- cashews
- chestnuts
- chia seeds
- coffee (daily)
- egg whites/ whole egg
- hazelnuts
- hemp
- macadamia nuts
- pecans
- pistachios
- poppy seeds
- pumpkin seeds
- sesame seeds
- sunflower seeds
- walnuts

CHAPTER FOUR

STAGE 2 RECIPES

HURRAH, I'M SO HAPPY to see you here in Stage 2! If you've made good progress with the Stage 1 reintroductions, it's a sign your body has done a significant amount of healing, so kudos to you. If you're still on the elimination phase or making your way through Stage 1, don't worry. There's no rush—the time for Stage 2 reintroductions will come. Until then, there are plenty of easily adaptable recipes here to fall in love with.

This stage sees egg whites as a reintroduction. Use them on their own to make the Maple Meringues (page 116). Or use the complete egg and enjoy a Scromelette (page 90). It's a hybrid of scrambled eggs and an omelet, and it's one of my favorites for breakfast or a light lunch. The beauty of having whole eggs in the diet is the speed with which you can make a cost-effective meal that's also highly nutritious, especially when you add some veggies or salad alongside. Do try the Sticky Toffee Pudding (page 113)—even if you feel you need to organize a dinner party to cook it.

Butter is a Stage 2 reintroduction and, when from a grass-fed source, rich in those fat-soluble vitamins that are so important for overall health.

Great for cooking, butter is incredible when melted over piping-hot steamed vegetables or an oven-baked sweet potato. And it is at its absolute finest in the Chicken Kiev (page 105). I used to love store-bought versions of this classic when I was younger, but now I find this healthier recipe much more satisfying.

Nuts and seeds are also brought back in this stage, opening up snack options and alternative dairy-free milks. Be sure to soak and sprout when possible, to extract antinutrients while unleashing nutrients that are essential for optimal function. Presoaking is strongly recommended for the best chance of tolerating these new foods. (See more in the Kitchen Basics section, page 10.)

Alcohol can be enjoyed in small quantities. Rather than challenging alcohol by the teaspoon method (page 35), you should slowly sip a small glassful of anything listed in the reintroduction table (page 30). Be certain that your drink is gluten-free and wait one week before repeating. Be sure to try the Rum 'n Raisin Stracciatella Ice Cream (page 114) in this chapter. It's a grown-up version of the one you enjoyed as a child, I'm willing to bet.

2

Chia seeds

AIP COMPLIANT See note.

FREEZER-FRIENDLY Yes

LOW FODMAP No

COCONUT-FREE Use a dairy-free seed/ nut milk or tigernut milk

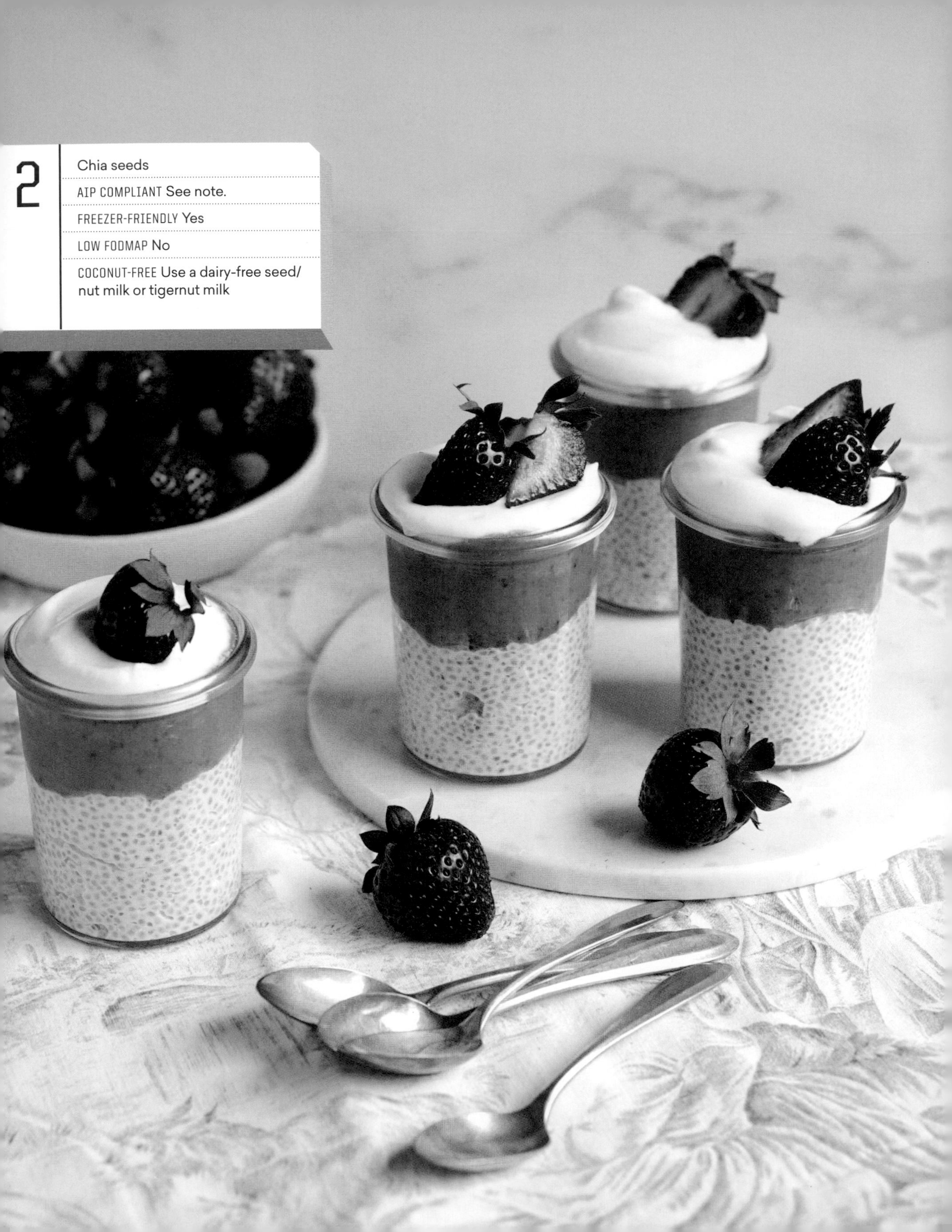

STRAWBERRY VANILLA
CHIA SEED PARFAIT

SERVES 2 TO 4,
DEPENDING ON
WHETHER IT'S
BREAKFAST
OR DESSERT

PREP TIME:
25 MINUTES,
PLUS SOAKING

CHIA BASE

1½ cups (375 ml)
coconut milk

½ cup (125 ml) filtered
water

⅓ cup (58.3 g) chia seeds

½ teaspoon alcohol-free
vanilla extract

1 teaspoon maple syrup
(optional)

Pinch sea salt

**STRAWBERRY
TOPPING**

2 cups (290 g)
strawberries, thawed if
previously frozen

1 avocado

1½ teaspoons (8 ml)
lemon juice

2 teaspoons (10 ml)
alcohol-free vanilla extract

Pinch sea salt

TO SERVE

Cooonut yogurt

Chia seeds are high in antioxidants and rich in omega-3 fatty acids, so they make a healthy breakfast or dessert. They are also a good source of soluble fiber. Always be sure to make the chia part several hours in advance so the seeds absorb the liquid in the bowl rather than absorb the liquid in your gut, possibly causing constipation.

To make the chia base, put the coconut milk, water, chia seeds, vanilla, maple syrup (if using), and salt in a medium bowl and mix together well. Cover and set aside in the refrigerator for at least 3 hours or overnight if possible, stirring once in a while.

To make the topping, put the strawberries, avocado, lemon juice, vanilla, and salt in your food processor. Blend until smooth and creamy.

To assemble, divide the chia mixture between four glasses or jars, and top with the strawberry mixture. Finish with a spoonful of coconut yogurt.

NOTE: **For a delicious AIP compliant smoothie, blend 2 cups strawberries, 1 cup (250 ml) coconut milk, ½ avocado, 1 teaspoon (5 ml) lemon juice, 1 teaspoon (5 ml) vanilla extract, a pinch of sea salt, 2 scoops grass-fed collagen (optional), ½ cup (125 ml) filtered water, and 3–4 large ice cubes. Makes 4 cups and serves 2 to 4.**

WATERCRESS SOUP
WITH QUICK PICKLED PEARS & TOASTED HAZELNUTS

SERVES 6 TO 8

PREP TIME: 45 MINUTES, PLUS PRESOAKING

COOK TIME: 45 MINUTES

PEARS

¾ cup (185 ml) white wine vinegar

1 tablespoon (15 ml) honey

1 large cinnamon stick, broken in two

4 whole cloves

¾ teaspoon coarse Himalayan pink salt

2 ripe but firm red pears, peeled, halved, cored, and sliced into 3 wedges each

SOUP

1 tablespoon (15 ml) extra virgin olive oil

1 leek, thinly sliced

2 cloves garlic, minced

1 lb (450 g) rutabaga, peeled and cut into 1-inch (2.5 cm) chunks

¾ lb (340 g) white sweet potato, peeled and cut into 1½-inch (3.5 cm) chunks

Pinch Himalayan pink salt

3 cups (750 ml) chicken broth

2 bunches watercress, roughly chopped

1 cup (60 g) chopped fresh flat-leaf parsley

2 tablespoons (30 ml) lemon juice

HAZELNUTS

½ cup (67.5 g) hazelnuts, soaked overnight

This is a great combination of flavors, and, if you're short on time, each part can be made in advance. The recipe makes more pickled pears than needed for the soup, so use them in salads, alongside liver paté, or on top of stews. They're extremely versatile. I used the red d'Anjou variety for this recipe, but Bartlett would also be lovely.

You will need a sterilized 1-pint (570 ml) jar.

To make the pears, put the vinegar, honey, cinnamon, cloves, and salt in a medium pan and stir. Bring slowly to a boil over medium heat. Put the pear slices in the sterilized jar and pour over the liquid and spices. Leave to cool; then cover the jar and store in the refrigerator until needed.

To make the soup, heat the oil in a large pan and add the leeks. Cook gently for 6 to 8 minutes until softened. Add the garlic and cook for 1 minute. Add the rutabaga and sweet potato, together with a pinch of salt, and combine. Stir in the broth and 2 cups (500 ml) filtered water, and bring to a simmer.

Cover the pan and cook for 25 to 30 minutes until the vegetables have softened. Add the watercress, parsley, and lemon juice and allow to wilt for a minute or two. Transfer the soup to a blender and blend until smooth. You will need to do this carefully in batches, or instead use an immersion blender. Taste and adjust the seasoning if needed.

Meanwhile, make the hazelnuts. Rinse the hazelnuts, place them in a clean tea towel and rub to remove the skins. Put a frying pan over medium heat and add the nuts. Cook for 5 minutes, shaking from time to time to stop them burning. Remove from the frying pan and put on a plate to cool.

Ladle the soup into large shallow bowls. Remove some pears from the pickling liquid and place on top of the soup. Roughly chop the toasted hazelnuts, scatter over the soup, and serve.

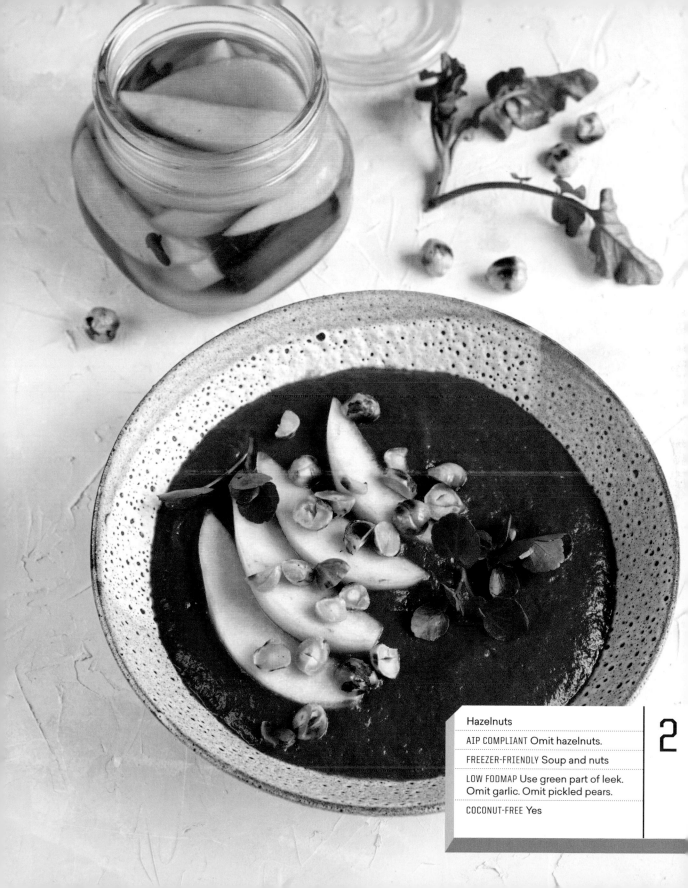

Hazelnuts

2

AIP COMPLIANT Omit hazelnuts.

FREEZER-FRIENDLY Soup and nuts

LOW FODMAP Use green part of leek.
Omit garlic. Omit pickled pears.

COCONUT-FREE Yes

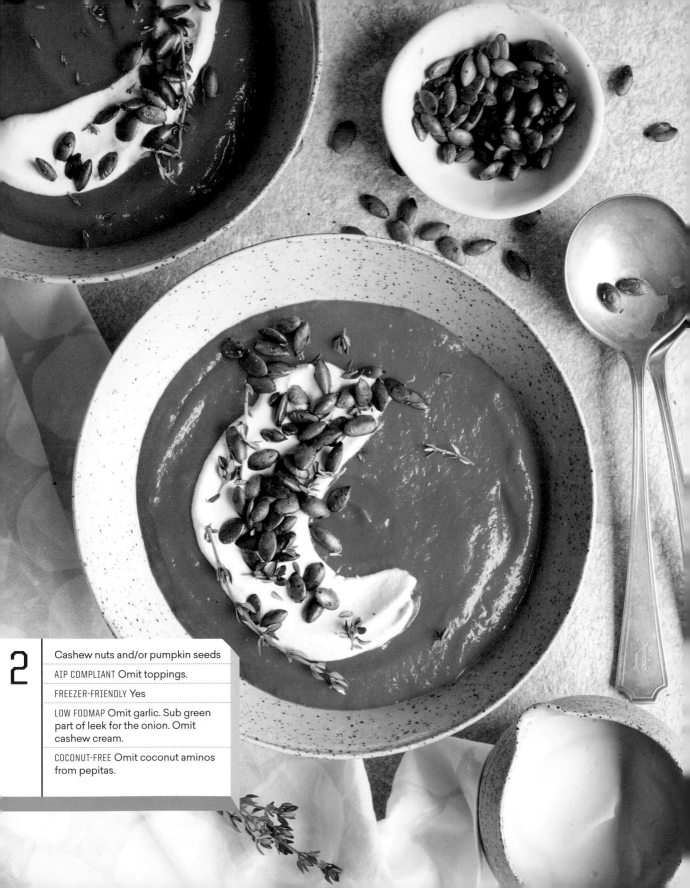

2

Cashew nuts and/or pumpkin seeds

AIP COMPLIANT Omit toppings.

FREEZER-FRIENDLY Yes

LOW FODMAP Omit garlic. Sub green part of leek for the onion. Omit cashew cream.

COCONUT-FREE Omit coconut aminos from pepitas.

ROASTED SWEET POTATO SOUP
WITH CASHEW CREAM & SESAME-TOASTED PEPITAS

SERVES 6

PREP TIME: 40 MINUTES, PLUS SOAKING

COOK TIME: 60 MINUTES

CASHEW CREAM

1 cup (5 oz) raw cashews, soaked for 6 hours

½–¾ cup (125–185 ml) filtered water

Pinch sea salt

PEPITAS

1 teaspoon (5 ml) coconut aminos

1 teaspoon (5 ml) sesame oil (Stage 1)

¾ cup (48 g) raw pumpkin seeds

Pinch sea salt

SOUP

3 lb (4 medium) sweet potatoes, peeled and cut into 1-inch (2.5 cm) pieces

1 large yellow onion, cut into 6–8 wedges

6 cloves garlic, unpeeled

4 tablespoons (60 ml) extra virgin olive oil, divided

3 stalks celery, thinly sliced

5–6 cups (1.3–1.5 L) chicken bone broth

2 sprigs fresh thyme

Pinch sea salt

I could never tire of soups—to me they are the definition of comfort food. Roasting the veggies first intensifies the flavors; then you add a silky-smooth cream topping and a pop of crunch from the pepitas. You can also use the cashew cream in sweet dishes, with the addition of a drizzle of maple syrup, and the pepitas make a great little snack on their own. Check the table on page 12 for how to prepare the pumpkin seeds.

To make the cashew cream, rinse the cashews and put in a blender, together with ½ cup (125 ml) of the water. Blend until smooth, scraping down the sides if necessary. Slowly add more water if needed, until it becomes the consistency of thick cream.

Preheat the oven to 375°F (190°C, or gas mark 5).

To make the pepitas, mix the coconut aminos and sesame oil together in a medium bowl and stir in the pumpkin seeds. Line a baking sheet with parchment paper and spread out the coated seeds. Place in the oven and toast for 12 to 14 minutes, stirring them halfway through the cooking time and keeping an eye on them so they don't burn. Remove and transfer to a large plate. When they're cool enough to try, have a taste and sprinkle over a little sea salt if desired. Allow to cool completely.

To make the soup, line a couple of large rimmed baking sheets with parchment paper and spread out the sweet potatoes, onion wedges, and garlic. Divide 3 tablespoons (45 ml) of the olive oil between each baking sheet and pop in the oven for 45 to 50 minutes, turning halfway through the cooking time. Remove from the oven and allow to cool.

Heat the remaining tablespoon of oil in a large saucepan and add the celery. Gently sauté for 6 minutes, or until softened. Squeeze the garlic flesh out of the casings and add to the pan, along with the sweet potato and onion. Pour in the broth, add the thyme and a pinch of salt, and bring to a simmer. Cook for 10 minutes until the sweet potatoes are completely tender.

Carefully transfer the soup in batches to a blender and blitz until smooth, or use an immersion blender to blend the soup in the saucepan. Taste and stir in more salt if needed. Pour into warm bowls and garnish with the cashew cream and toasted pepitas.

SCROMELETTE—
BEST EGGS EVER

SERVES 1

PREP TIME:
5 MINUTES

COOK TIME:
2 MINUTES

3 large pastured eggs

1½ teaspoons (8 ml) extra
virgin olive oil, bacon
grease, or fat of your
choice

¼–½ teaspoon herbes
de Provence

Pinch sea salt

A "scromelette" is our word for what is essentially a cross between scrambled eggs and an omelette. Spend a bit more time than usual to whisk your eggs as the extra air makes them super light and fluffy. Use a pan that can be heated while empty and your reward is the easiest egg pan you've ever cleaned!

Crack the eggs into a medium bowl, add the herbed de Provence and salt, and beat well.

Put a medium heavy-based pan over medium heat. When it's hot, add the cooking fat and swirl the pan to coat the base and a good ½ inch (1 cm) up the sides.

Return the pan to the heat and pour in the beaten eggs, which will sizzle as they hit the base. Resist the temptation to stir. Instead, leave for 30 seconds until you see the eggs start to cook up the sides of the pan.

With a wooden spoon, draw the eggs away from one side of the pan, allowing the excess liquid to fall back into the gap. Repeat several times until the eggs don't run back any more. Remove from the heat while the egg mixture is just undercooked as it will continue cooking.

Now turn out onto your plate, allowing the eggs to fold into a natural parcel.

I love to serve this with the dandelion-dulse relish (see page 57) and baby salad leaves.

2

Egg white (whole eggs)

AIP COMPLIANT No

FREEZER-FRIENDLY No

LOW FODMAP Yes

COCONUT-FREE Yes

ASIAN-STYLE SLAW
WITH SESAME SEEDS & TAMARIND DRESSING

SERVES 6

PREP TIME: 30 MINUTES

SALAD

8 oz (225 g) green papaya, peeled and cut into matchstick pieces

1 large carrot, cut into matchstick pieces

1 small red onion, thinly sliced

4 oz (110 g) Napa cabbage, finely shredded

6 oz (170 g) red cabbage, finely shredded

1 cup (16 g) chopped fresh cilantro

½ cup (20 g) fresh Thai basil, rolled and thinly sliced

⅓ cup (31.8 g) fresh mint leaves, chopped

1 tablespoon (8 g) white sesame seeds

DRESSING

1 garlic clove

1 lemongrass stalk, finely chopped

Zest of 1 large lime

1 tablespoon (15 ml) lime juice

2 teaspoons tamarind paste

1 teaspoon fish sauce

1 teaspoon coconut sugar

3 tablespoons (45 ml) avocado oil

3 tablespoons (45 ml) extra virgin olive oil

This is a very simple, refreshing salad that works with any type of protein. I also like to use this dressing over grilled chicken or fish, or just plain salad leaves. If you can't source green papaya, use a cucumber instead. If you don't have access to Thai basil, the regular type works well too.

To make the salad, put the papaya, carrot, onion, cabbage, cilantro, basil, mint, and sesame seeds in a large bowl.

To make the dressing, put the garlic, lemongrass, lime zest and juice, tamarind, fish sauce, sugar, and oils in a blender. Blend until smooth.

Pour the dressing over the salad, mix well, and serve.

Sesame seeds

AIP COMPLIANT Omit sesame seeds.

FREEZER-FRIENDLY No

LOW FODMAP Sub green part of a bunch of spring onions for onion. Omit garlic or use garlic oil instead of avocado oil.

COCONUT-FREE Omit coconut sugar.

2

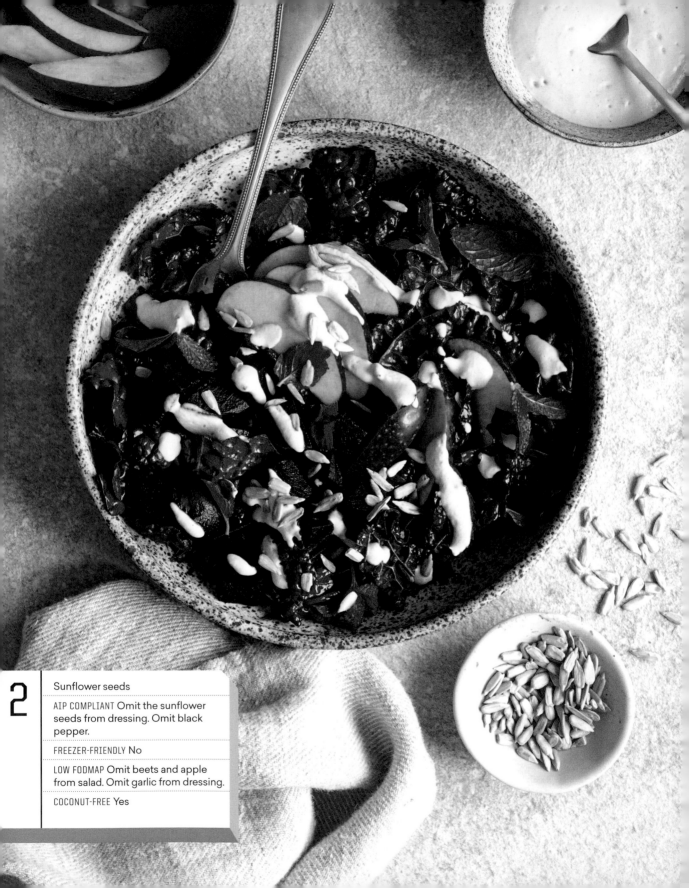

2 | Sunflower seeds

AIP COMPLIANT Omit the sunflower seeds from dressing. Omit black pepper.

FREEZER-FRIENDLY No

LOW FODMAP Omit beets and apple from salad. Omit garlic from dressing.

COCONUT-FREE Yes

KALE, BEET, APPLE SALAD
WITH SUNBUTTER DRESSING

SERVES 4 TO 6
AS A SIDE

PREP TIME:
20 MINUTES,
PLUS SOAKING

COOK TIME:
50 MINUTES

SALAD

12 oz (340 g) small beets

2 bunches lacinato kale,
chopped

1 teaspoon (5 ml) extra
virgin olive oil

½ cup (48 g) roughly
chopped fresh mint

1 crisp red apple such
as Pink Lady

DRESSING

⅓ cup (44.6 g) sunflower
seeds, soaked overnight,
drained, and rinsed

¼ cup (60 ml) plus
1 tablespoon (15 ml) extra
virgin olive oil

1 clove garlic

1 teaspoon (5 ml) lemon
juice

1 tablespoon (15 ml)
red wine vinegar

Pinch sea salt

Pinch black pepper
(Stage 1)

Massaging kale gives it a softer texture and less bitterness and makes it easier on your digestive system. Soak the sunflower seeds to make them easier to digest, too. If you like, you can sprout them in a couple of days. I don't ever use aluminum foil in my kitchen, which is a common way to cook beets for peeling. Instead I fit them snugly into a covered pan with a splash of water and oven bake until the skins slip off easily.

Preheat oven to 375°F (190°C, or gas mark 5).

To make the salad, wash the beets and give them a gentle scrub. Put them in a medium ovenproof lidded pan with a splash of water. Roast for 50 to 55 minutes until tender when pierced with a knife, turning halfway through the cooking time. Drain and set aside until they are cool enough to handle. Peel off the skins with your fingers, or scrape away with a small knife.

To make the salad, cut the central stalk from the kale leaves and discard. Shred the leaves and put in a large salad bowl. Add the oil and gently massage with clean hands for 3 to 4 minutes until the leaves have softened.

To make the dressing, put all the sunflower seeds, oil, garlic, lemon juice, vinegar, and a pinch of salt and pepper in a blender with 2 tablespoons (30 ml) filtered water. Blend until smooth.

Cut the beets into bite-size pieces. Cut the apple into quarters, remove the core, and cut each quarter into 4 slices. Add these to the kale, together with the mint.

Add the dressing, give the salad a toss, and serve.

ELEGANT
WHITE SALAD

SERVES 4

PREP TIME:
25 MINUTES

SALAD

1 large fennel bulb and fronds, thinly sliced

3-inch (7.5 cm) piece daikon, thinly sliced

2 stalks celery, thinly sliced

3 scallions, thinly sliced on the diagonal

Small handful kumquats, sliced

1 small endive, base cut off and leaves separated

½ cup (15 g) microgreens

½ cup (60 g) roughly chopped walnuts, soaked and dehydrated

DRESSING

1 teaspoon (5 ml) lemon juice

2 tablespoons (30 ml) extra virgin olive oil

1 tablespoon (15 ml) white wine vinegar

Pinch Himalayan pink salt

Pinch white pepper
(Stage 1)

This delicate salad is at its best when served with oily fish such as sardines, mackerel, or salmon. It's also wonderful alongside fresh crab or shrimp. If you can't find kumquats, substitute with segments from a small blood orange. A couple of sliced plums would also work well. Don't forget that nuts are always more digestible when soaked and dehydrated first. See page 12 for more information.

To make the salad, assemble the fennel, daikon, celery, scallions, kumquats, endive, microgreens, and walnuts in a serving bowl or on a platter.

To make the dressing, whisk together the lemon juice, oil, vinegar, salt, and pepper.

Pour the dressing over the salad, and serve.

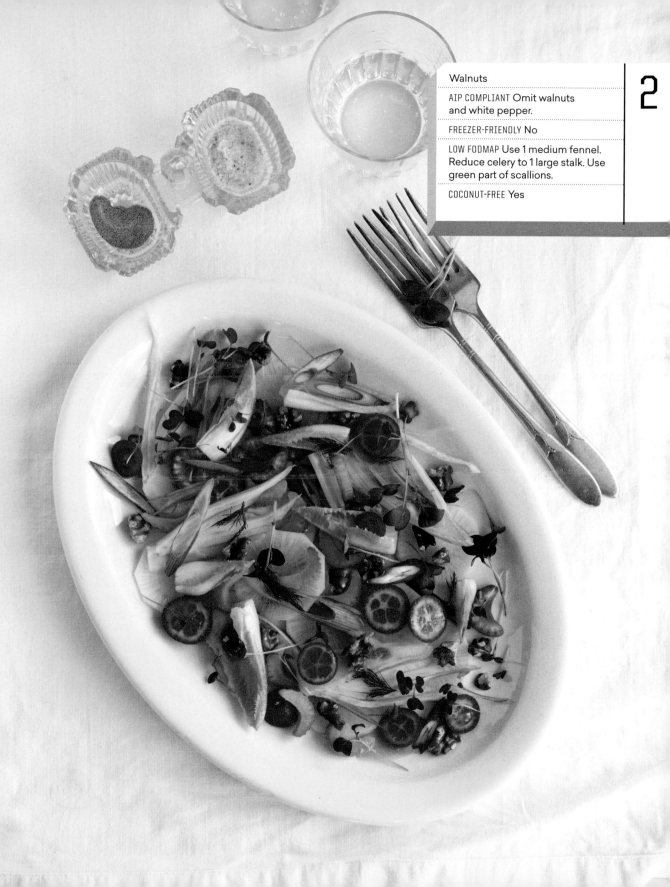

Walnuts

AIP COMPLIANT Omit walnuts and white pepper.

FREEZER-FRIENDLY No

LOW FODMAP Use 1 medium fennel. Reduce celery to 1 large stalk. Use green part of scallions.

COCONUT-FREE Yes

2

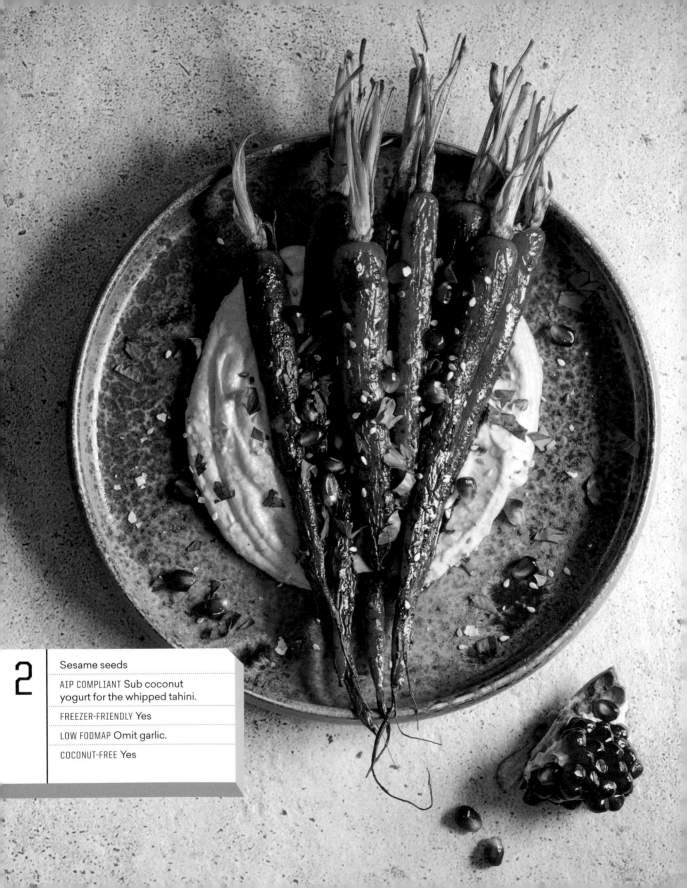

2

Sesame seeds

AIP COMPLIANT Sub coconut yogurt for the whipped tahini.

FREEZER-FRIENDLY Yes

LOW FODMAP Omit garlic.

COCONUT-FREE Yes

ROASTED POMEGRANATE CARROTS

ON WHIPPED TAHINI

SERVES 4 AS A SIDE

PREP TIME: 45 MINUTES

COOK TIME: 30 MINUTES

CARROTS

1 cup (250 ml) pure pomegranate juice

1 tablespoon (20 g) molasses

2 teaspoons (10 ml) lemon juice

16 equal-sized carrots, trimmed

1 tablespoon (15 ml) extra virgin olive oil

½ teaspoon ground cinnamon

Pinch flaky sea salt

2 tablespoons (16 g) sesame seeds

Small handful pomegranate seeds

¼ cup (15 g) chopped fresh flat-leaf parsley

WHIPPED TAHINI (MAKES 1½ CUPS)

1 cup (240 g) tahini

2 cloves garlic, minced

2 tablespoons (30 ml) lemon juice

Pinch sea salt

¾ cup (185 ml) cold filtered water

It has to be said, roasted carrots are sweet and delicious enough on their own. But when you brush them with pomegranate molasses, they become something very special. Store-bought pomegranate molasses is heavy on sugar, but the good news is it's very simple to make your own. My recipe uses blackstrap molasses, which boasts an impressive list of nutrients so the end result is a rich and far healthier version.

Preheat the oven to 400°F (200°C, or gas mark 6).

To make the carrots, put the pomegranate juice, molasses, and lemon juice in a small pan and bring to a boil. Turn down to simmer and cook for 30 minutes, or until reduced to ¼ cup (60 ml). Set aside to cool and thicken.

Scrub the carrots, halve if they are large, and put in a large bowl. Drizzle over the oil and toss to coat. Arrange on a large rimmed baking sheet, leaving a space between each one so they roast rather than steam. Sprinkle over the cinnamon and place in the oven for 15 minutes.

Remove the carrots and brush with a thin layer of pomegranate syrup. Return to the oven for 10 to 15 minutes until golden brown and tender. Remove from the oven and sprinkle with flaky salt.

While the carrots are cooking, make the whipped tahini. Put the tahini, garlic, lemon juice, and sea salt in the small bowl of your food processor, fitted with the S blade. Turn the motor on and slowly drizzle in enough water to achieve the consistency of thickened, fluffy mayonnaise. Taste and adjust the flavoring to your liking.

Divide the tahini between four plates and arrange the carrots over the top. Garnish with the sesame seeds, pomegranates, and parsley.

CREPES WITH SHRIMP

MAKES 8

PREP TIME: 30 MINUTES,
PLUS SOAKING

COOK TIME: 35 MINUTES

CREPES

1 tablespoon (8 g) sesame seeds,
soaked and dried

⅓ cup (44 g) tapioca flour

½ teaspoon ground turmeric

¼ cup (60 ml) coconut milk

Pinch sea salt

2 cups (100 g) beansprouts
(Stage 1)

Avocado or coconut oil

5 scallions, thinly sliced

¾ lb (340 g) cooked, peeled
small shrimp

DIPPING SAUCE

4 teaspoons fish sauce

4 cloves garlic, minced

4 tablespoons (60 ml) coconut
aminos

2 tablespoons (30 ml) raw apple
cider vinegar

4 tablespoons (60 ml) sesame oil
(Stage 1)

1 teaspoon coconut sugar

TO SERVE

½ head lettuce, leaves separated

Small handful fresh cilantro

Small handful fresh Thai basil

Small handful fresh mint

Lime wedges

Based on the Vietnamese Bánh xèo, these savory sizzling crepes are a favorite street snack. They often include pork, so you could use leftover pork belly (page 62) in addition to—or instead of—the shrimp. Traditionally they are wrapped in a lettuce leaf with an assortment of herbs, and dipped into Nuoc Cham, a sweet-sour sauce. Sesame is not necessarily a traditional component of this recipe, but it is common in Vietnamese cuisine—and a tasty way of incorporating if you have reintroduced it. For information on preparing sesame seeds, see page 12 in Kitchen Basics.

Toast the sesame seeds in a dry frying pan until golden, and set aside.

To make the dipping sauce, add the fish sauce, garlic, coconut aminos, apple cider vinegar, oil, and sugar to a small bowl and mix well. Set aside.

Put the tapioca flour and turmeric in a medium bowl. Pour in the coconut milk and ¼ cup (60 ml) water and whisk to a smooth, runny batter.

Divide the scallions, shrimp, and beansprouts into 8 portions.

Put the frying pan over medium heat. Put 1 teaspoon (5 ml) of the oil in the pan and add a portion of the spring onions and shrimp. Pour ¼ cup of the batter over and around and add a sprinkling of sesame seeds and some beansprouts. Cover the pan and cook for 2 minutes; then remove the lid and cook for 2 minutes, regulating the temperature as necessary.

Fold the crepe and move to a warm plate. Make the other crepes in the same way.

The traditional way to eat these is to tear the crepes into bite-sized pieces, wrap in a lettuce leaf with a selection of herbs, and dip into the dipping sauce. Serve the lime wedges on the side

NOTE **If you have reintroduced rice, a more authentic batter is ¼ cup (45 g) white rice flour, ¼ cup (60 ml) coconut milk, and ¼ cup (60 ml) water.**

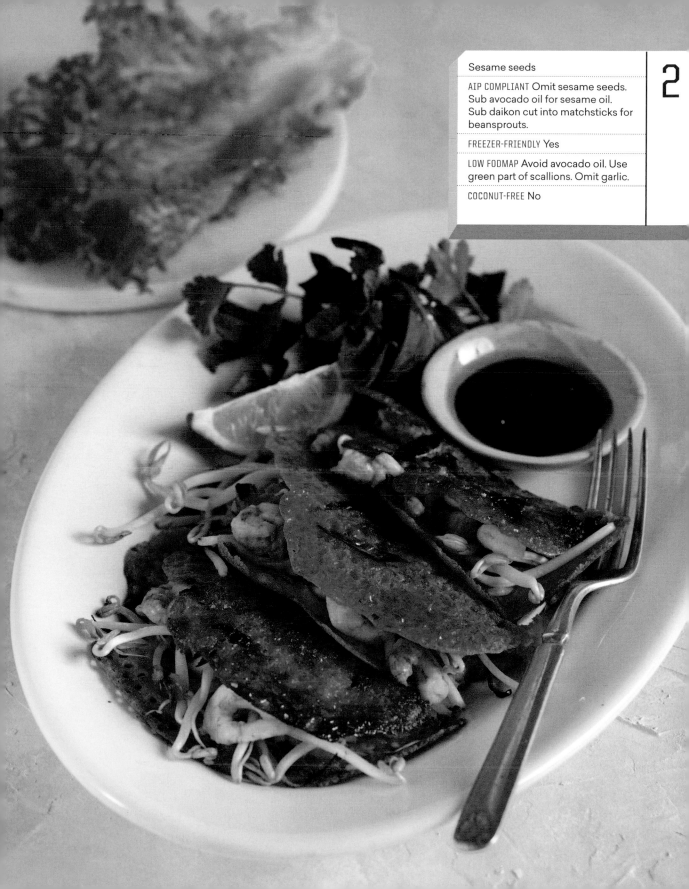

Sesame seeds

AIP COMPLIANT Omit sesame seeds. Sub avocado oil for sesame oil. Sub daikon cut into matchsticks for beansprouts.

FREEZER-FRIENDLY Yes

LOW FODMAP Avoid avocado oil. Use green part of scallions. Omit garlic.

COCONUT-FREE No

2

SEED-CRUSTED SALMON
ON HERBED CAULI RICE

SERVES 4

PREP TIME: 30 MINUTES,
PLUS SOAKING

COOK TIME: 10 MINUTES

SALMON

2 tablespoons (20 g)
sunflower seeds

2 tablespoons (20 g)
pumpkin seeds

2 tablespoons (16 g) white
sesame seeds

2 tablespoons (14 g) hemp
seeds

2 tablespoons (16.5 g)
tapioca flour

2 tablespoons (30 ml) extra
virgin olive oil, divided

4 salmon fillets, skinless

CAULI RICE

1 tablespoon (15 ml) extra
virgin olive oil

1 medium head cauliflower,
riced

½ cup (30 g) chopped fresh
flat-leaf parsley

¼ cup (16 g) chopped
fresh dill

½ cup (8 g) chopped fresh
cilantro

Pinch sea salt

Pinch black pepper
(Stage 1)

4 lemon wedges

This crunchy topping works really well with salmon because it complements its flavor rather than dominating it. Keep an eye on the salmon as it's cooking because it will be bitter if the seeds are scorched. Cauliflower is one of the most versatile vegetables and makes a wonderful substitute for rice. I like to add in handfuls of herbs for color and added nutrients. See page 12 for how to soak and dry the seeds.

To make the salmon, lightly crush the sunflower and pumpkins seeds using a mortar and pestle. Stir in the sesame and hemp seeds and tip onto a large plate. Put the tapioca flour on a second plate and 1 tablespoon (15 ml) of the olive oil on a third.

Coat each salmon fillet with the tapioca flour and pat to dust off the excess. Place the fillets in the olive oil for a light coating, then press them into the seeds and coat both sides.

To make the cauli rice, put a large sauté pan over medium heat and add 1 tablespoon (15 ml) olive oil. Tip in the riced cauliflower and sauté for 3 to 4 minutes, or until tender. Remove from the heat and toss in the herbs. Season to taste.

Meanwhile, heat a large frying pan over low-medium and add 1 tablespoon (15 ml) olive oil. When the pan is hot, add the fish, presentation side down, making sure the fillets don't touch each other or they will steam. Cook for 2 minutes; then turn the fillets over and cook for 2 minutes or so more, regulating the temperature so the seeds don't burn. The seeds should be golden brown and the salmon just cooked through.

To serve, divide the cauliflower rice between four plates. Arrange the salmon on top and place a lemon wedge to one side.

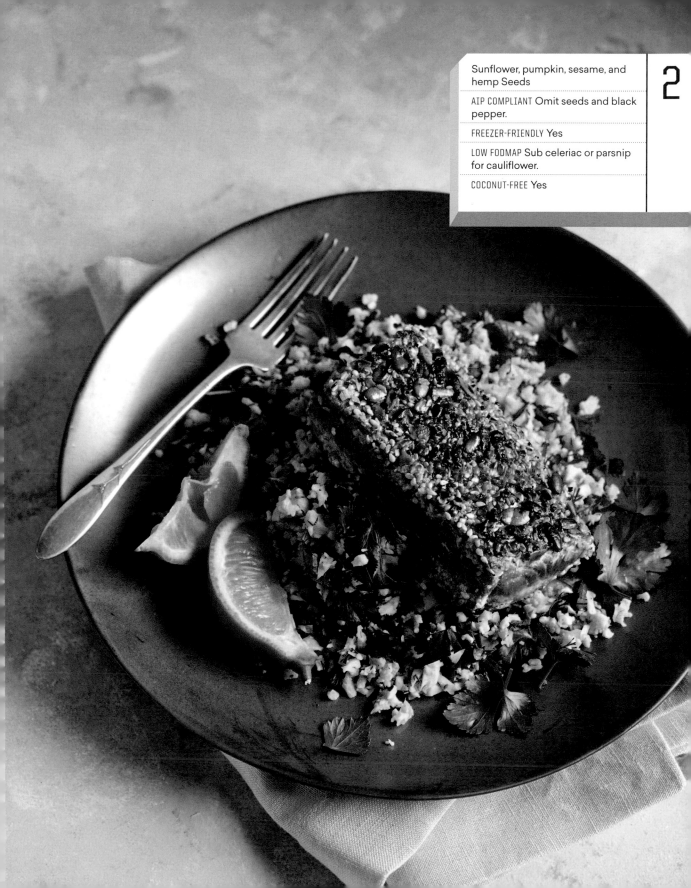

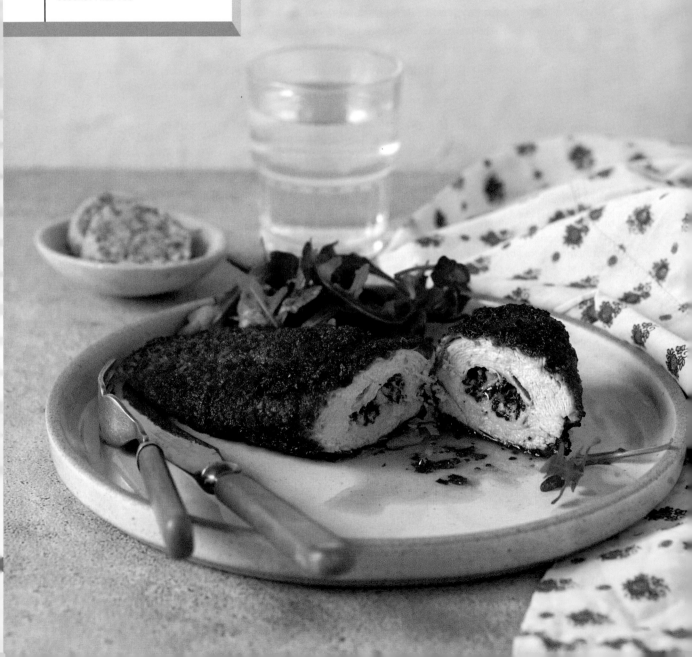

2

Sunflower, pumpkin, sesame, and hemp seeds

AIP COMPLIANT Omit seeds and black pepper.

FREEZER-FRIENDLY Yes

LOW FODMAP Sub celeriac or parsnip for cauliflower.

COCONUT-FREE Yes

CHICKEN KIEV

SERVES 4

PREP TIME:
40 MINUTES,
PLUS CHILLING

COOK TIME:
30 MINUTES

4 oz (110 g) unsalted grass-fed butter, softened

6 cloves garlic, minced

¼ cup (15 g) finely packed chopped fresh curly parsley

½ teaspoon sea salt

4 pastured, skinless, boneless chicken breasts

3 tablespoons (25 g) tapioca flour

6 oz (3 cups) plantain chips, ground to a fine breadcrumb consistency (1½ cups)

2 eggs

Extra virgin olive oil to fry

A bag of plantain chips has never been put to better use: Blitzed in the food processor, they become a wonderfully crunchy substitute for panko breadcrumbs. If you can't source plantain chips, sweet potato chips will also do the job. I like to keep a supply of garlic butter in the freezer for livening up steamed veggies or zucchini noodles. Having a ready supply also makes this a speedy but fun meal that everyone will enjoy.

Preheat the oven to 400°F (200°C, or gas mark 6).

Mix the butter, garlic, parsley, and sea salt in a small bowl. Place on a piece of parchment paper and roll to form a log. Twist either end like a cracker and refrigerate until firm.

Cut a 1-inch (2.5 cm) slit into the center of the thick end of each chicken breast and push the knife down to create a deep cavity. Be careful not to pierce through to the outer skin. Divide the garlic butter between each chicken breast and push down into the cavity. Remove part of the small fillet attached to the chicken and push this into the cavity to form a plug, so the butter doesn't run out.

Put the flour and plantain chips onto separate plates. Whisk the eggs in a shallow bowl.

Dip the chicken in the flour, dust off the excess, and then dip in the eggs. Now put the chicken in the plantain crumbs and coat well. Set aside on a large plate.

Heat the olive oil in a large, ovenproof frying pan. Add the chicken to the pan. Don't overcrowd or they'll steam rather than brown. Fry the chicken until golden brown all over, 2 to 3 minutes each side; then pop in the oven for 20 to 25 minutes until cooked through. The exact timing will depend on the size of the chicken pieces.

BONED CHICKEN
STUFFED WITH PISTACHIOS & FIGS

SERVES 6

PREP TIME:
30 MINUTES

COOK TIME:
90 MINUTES

3 dried figs

1 tablespoon (15 ml)
extra virgin olive oil

1 medium shallot, finely
chopped

½ lb (225 g) ground pork

3 asparagus spears, sliced

¼ cup (31 g) pistachios,
soaked overnight and
dehydrated

1 tablespoon (4 g) chopped
fresh tarragon

1 tablespoon (6 g) chopped
fresh mint

2 tablespoons (8 g)
chopped fresh flat-leaf
parsley

Pinch salt

Pinch black pepper
(Stage 1)

3 lb (1.4 kg) pasture-raised
chicken, boned completely

Boning out a chicken takes me back to my culinary days when we had to bone and stuff a small chicken for our final exam. I boned one every day for two weeks and got the timing down from twenty minutes to two. Have your butcher bone out the entire bird, leaving the skin intact; this will keep your stuffing inside when you wrap it up. Remember to keep the bones for making broth.

You will need some poultry lacers or cocktail sticks.

Preheat the oven to 400°F (200°C, or gas mark 6).

Make the stuffing: Plump the figs in hot water for 20 minutes. Drain, chop, and leave on a plate to cool. Put the oil in a small pan and gently cook the shallot until softened. Remove from the heat, tip onto a plate, and allow to cool.

In a large bowl, mix the ground pork with the asparagus, pistachios, tarragon, mint, parsley, salt, and pepper (if using).

Lay out the chicken on a board, skin side down. Spoon the stuffing in the middle and wrap up the chicken tightly, using several poultry lacers or cocktail sticks to secure.

Place the chicken on a wire rack over a roasting pan, seam side down, and bake for 90 minutes, basting mid way, until the juices run clear when pierced with a skewer.

Transfer to a board and allow to rest for 20 minutes. Serve hot or cold.

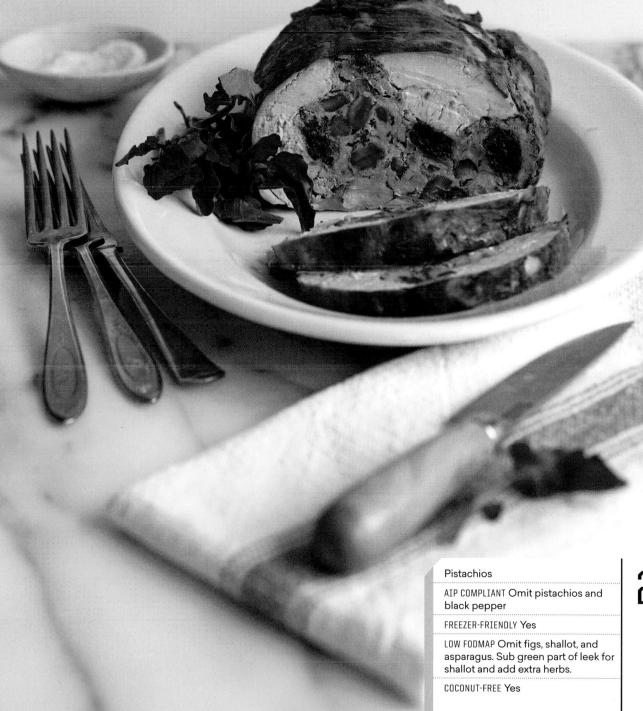

Pistachios	**2**
AIP COMPLIANT Omit pistachios and black pepper	
FREEZER-FRIENDLY Yes	
LOW FODMAP Omit figs, shallot, and asparagus. Sub green part of leek for shallot and add extra herbs.	
COCONUT-FREE Yes	

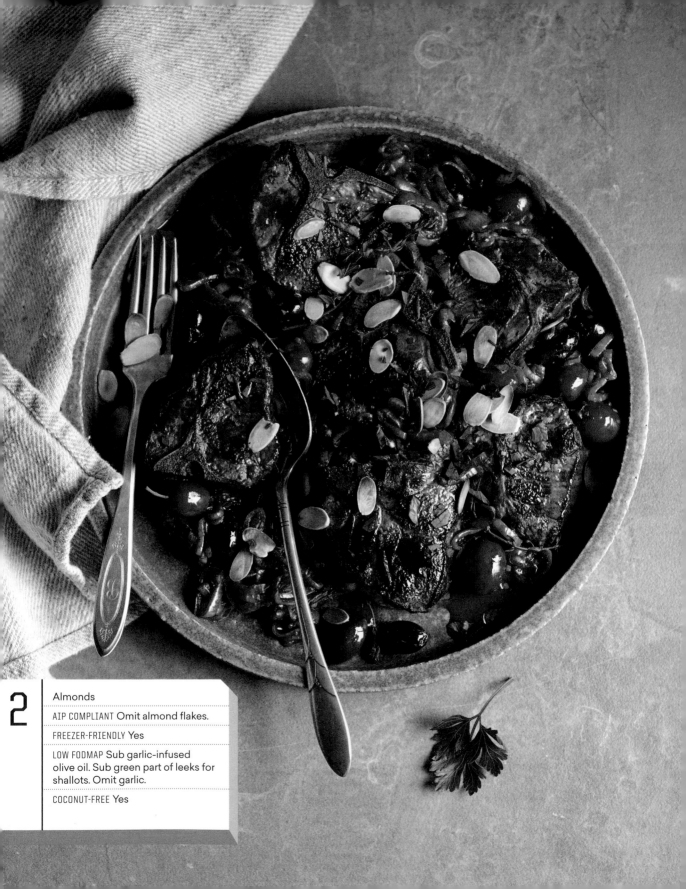

2

Almonds

AIP COMPLIANT Omit almond flakes.

FREEZER-FRIENDLY Yes

LOW FODMAP Sub garlic-infused olive oil. Sub green part of leeks for shallots. Omit garlic.

COCONUT-FREE Yes

SPANISH LAMB CHOPS
WITH SAFFRON & ALMONDS

SERVES 4

PREP TIME:
20 MINUTES,
PLUS SOAKING AND
MARINATING

COOK TIME:
25 MINUTES

6–8 thick lamb loin chops

3 tablespoons (45 ml)
extra virgin olive oil

3 large sprigs fresh thyme

3 tablespoons silvered
almonds, soaked and dried

6 small/medium shallots,
sliced

4 large cloves garlic,
minced

⅓ cup (80 ml) sherry
vinegar

½ cup (50 g) green olives

½ cup (50 g) black olives

½ cup (125 ml) rich chicken
bone broth

⅛ teaspoon saffron
stamens

2 tablespoons (8 g) finely
chopped fresh flat-leaf
parsley

Almonds have many benefits in our diet. They are high in key nutrients that support healthy brain function and help control blood sugar regulation. However, most nuts are high in omega-6, which, when eaten too often and in large quantities, may contribute to inflammation. The saying "everything in moderation" definitely applies when eating them, so moderation is what you get in this recipe. See page 12 for how to prepare the almonds.

Put the lamb chops in a shallow dish and add the oil and thyme sprigs. Turn the lamb over to coat, cover, and leave to marinate in the fridge for at least an hour, overnight if possible.

When you're ready to cook, remove lamb chops from the fridge and allow them to come to room temperature.

Put a heavy-based frying pan over medium heat and, when hot, add the slivered almonds. Toast for a minute or so until golden, shaking the pan frequently to avoid burning. Transfer to a cold plate to stop them cooking further.

Stack the chops together and place them fat edge down in the pan until browned along the edges. This allows the fat to render down into the pan. Then lay the chops down and cook for 3 minutes each side, depending on how thick they are and what degree of doneness you prefer. Remove the lamb and keep warm.

Add the shallots and garlic to the pan, lower the heat, and cook for 5 minutes or until softened. Add a little oil to the pan if it looks dry. Raise the heat to medium again and pour in the sherry vinegar, scraping up any sediment and incorporating it into the pan to add flavor. Add the olives, broth, saffron, and lamb juices. Bring to a simmer and allow to bubble for 2 minutes, or until the liquid has reduced by half.

Put the lamb chops onto plates and spoon the sauce around. Scatter the parsley and toasted almonds over the top, and serve.

BEEF & CHESTNUT
STEW

SERVES 6

PREP TIME: 30 MINUTES

COOK TIME: 3 HOURS

2 tablespoons (30 ml) extra virgin olive oil, divided

2¼ lb (1 kg) boneless grass-fed beef chuck steak, cut into 1½-inch (3.5 cm) cubes

2 medium red onions, thinly sliced

2 large stalks celery, thinly sliced

7 oz (200 g) brown mushrooms, sliced

5 slices bacon, chopped

4 cloves garlic, minced

1 teaspoon ground cinnamon

5 whole cloves

¼ cup (60 ml) sherry vinegar

2 bay leaves

3 long sprigs fresh thyme

3 cups (750 ml) rich beef bone broth

Pared rind and ⅓ cup (80 ml) fresh orange juice

Pinch sea salt

Pinch black pepper (Stage 1)

1¼ cups (7 oz) cooked chestnuts

I absolutely love stews. Chestnuts are a wonderful addition to this stew, which is rich and full of flavor, perfect for a cool night or lazy weekend lunch. I buy my chestnuts ready-cooked in small bags at the grocery store; they're fairly inexpensive. You can easily make this stew a day or two before serving as it reheats really well and tastes just as amazing.

Preheat the oven to 300°F (150°C, or gas mark 2).

Heat 1 tablespoon (15 ml) of the oil in a large Dutch oven over medium-high heat. Brown the meat in batches, remove to a plate, and set aside.

Add the second tablespoon of oil to the now empty pan. Tip in the onions and stir them around the base, scraping up as much sediment as you can as the onions release their juices. This adds color as well as flavor.

Turn the heat down to low and sweat the onions for 6 to 8 minutes until translucent. If your pan becomes too brown and parched, add a tablespoon of water.

Now add the celery, mushrooms, and bacon to the pan. Raise the heat to medium and cook for 6 to 7 minutes until softened. Stir in the garlic, cinnamon, and cloves, and cook for 1 to 2 minutes.

Pour in the sherry vinegar and deglaze the pan, scraping the sediment and stirring until the vinegar has evaporated. Return the browned meat to the pan, together with the bay leaves, thyme, broth, orange rind, and juice. Add salt and pepper, if using. Mix well, making sure the meat is covered by the liquid. Bring the stew to a boil, cover, and place in the oven.

Cook for 2½ hours, or until the meat is tender. Check halfway through the cooking time to make sure the stew isn't drying out and top up with extra broth or water if needed. Stir in the chestnuts and cook for 15 minutes.

Remove from the oven, adjust the seasonings if needed, and serve immediately. This pairs well with the parsnip purée on page 59 and simply sautéed greens.

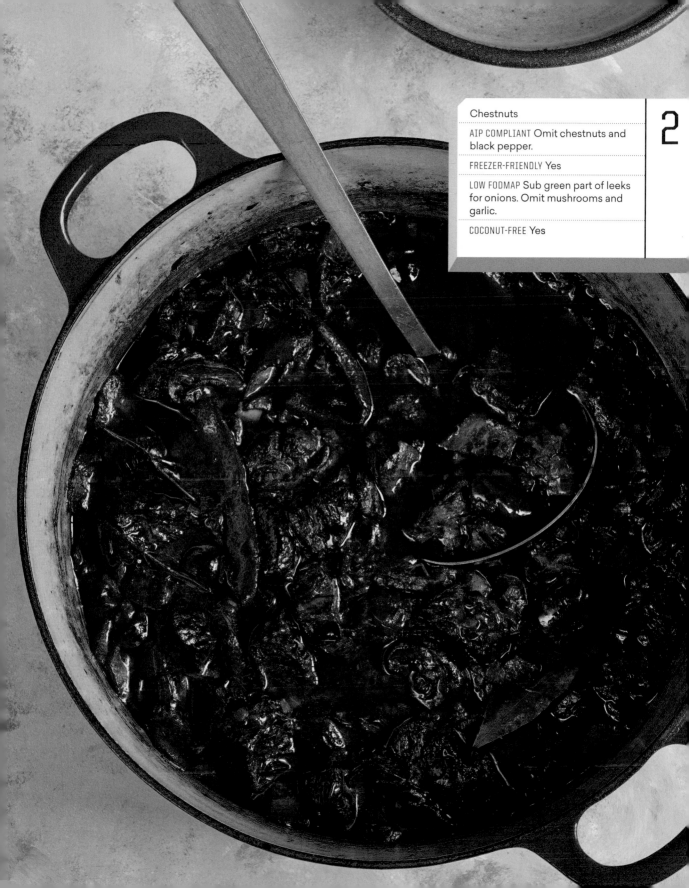

Chestnuts

AIP COMPLIANT Omit chestnuts and black pepper.

FREEZER-FRIENDLY Yes

LOW FODMAP Sub green part of leeks for onions. Omit mushrooms and garlic.

COCONUT-FREE Yes

2

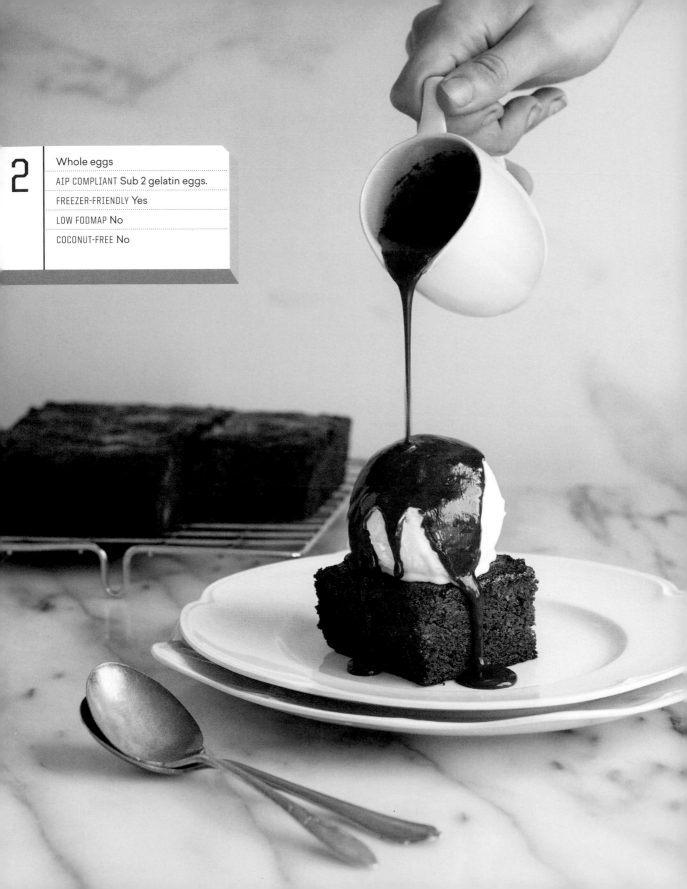

2

Whole eggs

AIP COMPLIANT Sub 2 gelatin eggs.

FREEZER-FRIENDLY Yes

LOW FODMAP No

COCONUT-FREE No

STICKY TOFFEE PUDDING

SERVES 10+

PREP TIME:
25 MINUTES, PLUS
STANDING TIME

COOK TIME:
60 MINUTES

PUDDING

10 dates, pits removed

1 teaspoon bicarbonate
of soda

½ cup (100 g) softened lard

3 tablespoons (24 g)
coconut sugar

2 large eggs

1 cup (110 g) tigernut flour

¼ cup (35 g) coconut flour

¼ cup (33 g) arrowroot
starch

Pinch sea salt

SAUCE (MAKES 1 CUP)

1 can (2 cups (250 ml))
coconut milk

3 tablespoons (24 g)
coconut sugar

1 tablespoon (15 ml)
blackstrap molasses

2 tablespoons (30 ml)
coconut oil

Pinch sea salt

For a very special, every-so-often treat, look no further than my take on one of Britain's finest. My husband—who always appreciates a good cake—tells me this recipe alone is worth the cost of this book! Be warned though, a little goes a long way. If you haven't reintroduced eggs, use two gelatin eggs instead (page 11). I serve this with vanilla ice cream—just follow the recipe for Rum 'n Raisin Stracciatella Ice Cream (page 114), omitting the rum, raisins and cacao.

Place a baking sheet in the oven on the middle shelf and preheat to 350°F (175°C, or gas mark 4). Line a 7-inch (18 cm) square tin with parchment paper.

To make the pudding, put the pitted dates in a medium pan and pour over ½ pint (290 ml) of water. Bring to a boil, remove from the heat, and stir in the bicarbonate of soda. Set aside for 30 minutes.

Put the lard in your mixer bowl and add the coconut sugar. Mix until pale and creamy.

Break the eggs in a small bowl and mix briefly with a fork or small whisk. Add to the mixing bowl in stages, with the motor running.

Sift in the flours, arrowroot, salt, and combine. If you are using gelatin eggs, make and add them here (see page 11 in Kitchen Basics). Tip in the dates, together with all the liquid, and give it all a thorough mix.

Put the mixture in the lined tin and place in the oven, on top of the baking sheet. Bake for 40 minutes until firm to the touch and coming away from the sides of the parchment.

Meanwhile, make the sauce. Put the coconut milk, sugar, molasses, oil, and salt in a medium pan. Bring to a simmer and cook, stirring occasionally, for 30 to 35 minutes until it coats the back of a spoon. It will firm up as it cools.

Pour 2 to 3 tablespoons (30 to 45 ml) of sauce over the cake and pop it back in the oven for 3 to 4 minutes to allow the sauce to seep in. Pour the remaining sauce into a jug to pass at the table.

This sauce is also amazing as a topping for homemade ice cream or yogurt.

RUM 'N RAISIN
STRACCIATELLA ICE CREAM

SERVES 8

PREP TIME:
40 MINUTES,
PLUS SOAKING
AND CHILLING

½ cup (72.5 g) uncoated
raisins

½ cup (125 ml) gluten-free
rum

2½ cups (625 ml) coconut
milk, refrigerated

3 tablespoons (45 ml)
maple syrup

1 teaspoon (5 ml) vanilla
extract

Pinch sea salt

3½ tablespoons raw cacao
(Stage 1)

4 tablespoons (60 ml)
melted coconut oil

There are so many possibilities with this ice cream, depending on where you are in your reintroductions, your flavor preferences, and the taste buds of the people with whom you are sharing. Make this as a Rum 'n Raisin, or maybe just a Stracciatella, because they're really two different ice creams rolled into one. In the spirit of indulgence, I guarantee you won't regret committing to the recipe in its entirety.

You will need a plain piping bag or a strong resealable plastic bag with a small hole cut in the corner. For best results, you will also need an ice cream machine.

Put the raisins in a small bowl and pour over the rum to cover. Set aside for at least 4 hours, even overnight. The longer the raisins soak, the stronger they'll be.

Stir the coconut milk, maple syrup, vanilla, and sea salt in a jug. Drain the raisins, reserving 1 tablespoon (15 ml) of the rum and add to the jug. Pour into the ice cream bowl and churn, following the manufacturer's instructions.

Stir the cacao powder into the melted coconut oil in stages, to avoid lumps. Set aside.

Once the mixture is nearly ready, put the chocolate mixture in the piping bag. While the ice cream machine is moving, slowly pipe in the chocolate mixture. It will harden into shards on impact. You may have more chocolate than you need.

Transfer the ice cream to a freezer-proof container and place in the freezer to firm up before serving.

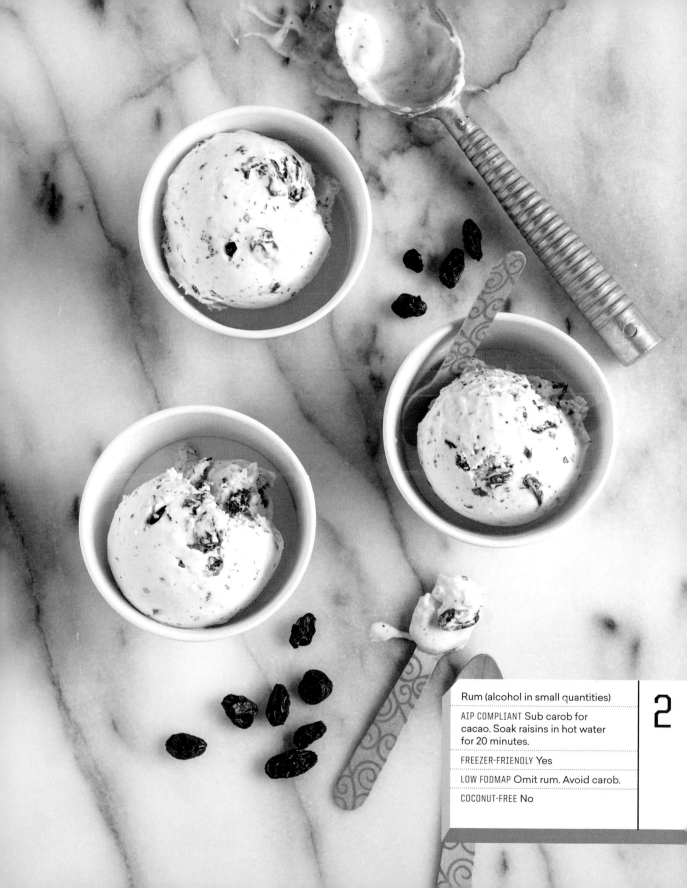

Rum (alcohol in small quantities)

AIP COMPLIANT Sub carob for cacao. Soak raisins in hot water for 20 minutes.

FREEZER-FRIENDLY Yes

LOW FODMAP Omit rum. Avoid carob.

COCONUT-FREE No

2

MAPLE MERINGUES
WITH VINEGAR-INFUSED BERRIES

MAKES 10 TO 12

PREP TIME:
15 MINUTES

COOK TIME: 2 HOURS,
PLUS 3 HOURS COOLING

MERINGUES

3 large egg whites

Pinch fine sea salt

Pinch cream of tartar

½ cup (161 g) maple syrup

BERRIES

6 oz (170 g) fresh
blackberries

6 oz (170 g) fresh
raspberries

Juice of ½ orange

1 tablespoon (15 ml) raw
apple cider vinegar

Berries are Paleolithic man's antioxidant, and they are amazing macerated in apple cider vinegar for a little acidic zing. They work really well with the sweetness of the maple meringues. I also love making mini meringues to eat with Choco-Hazelnut Hummus (page 163). Don't forget to save the yolks for Mint Mayonnaise (page 81).

Preheat the oven to 225°F (110°C, or gas mark ½). Line 2 to 3 flat baking sheets with parchment paper and set aside.

Wipe a cut lemon (or small amount of vinegar) around your mixing bowl and your whisk, and wipe dry. This ensures the bowl is clean and won't affect the volume of your egg whites.

To make the meringues, put the egg whites in the clean bowl with the salt and cream of tartar and whisk until stiff. Next, add the maple syrup in a slow, steady stream while whisking, until the mixture is very stiff and shiny.

Spoon heaped tablespoons of the mixture onto the parchment paper and bake for 2 hours. Turn the oven off and leave the meringues inside to cool down completely for at least 3 hours, even overnight.

Meanwhile, make the berries. Put the blackberries, raspberries, orange juice, and apple cider vinegar in a medium bowl. Mix together well, crushing slightly with a spoon. Set aside to infuse.

To serve, place a meringue on a plate with a spoonful of the vinegar-infused berries on the side.

2

Egg whites

AIP COMPLIANT Omit meringues.

FREEZER-FRIENDLY Yes

LOW FODMAP Sub strawberries for
blackberries.

COCONUT-FREE Yes

APPLE & WALNUT CRUMBLE
WITH ROSE-SCENTED CREAM

SERVES 6

PREP TIME:
30 MINUTES

COOK TIME:
55 MINUTES

CRUMBLE

2 tablespoons (30 ml)
lemon juice

5 apples of mixed varieties,
peeled and cored

¾ teaspoon ground
cinnamon

2 tablespoons (18 g) and
2 teaspoons (6 g) coconut
sugar, divided

½ cup (76 g) cassava flour

½ cup (55 g) tigernut flour

Pinch sea salt

4 oz (110 g) cold leaf lard

½ cup (60 g) walnut pieces,
soaked and dehydrated

CREAM

1½ cups (a 400 ml can)
coconut cream

2 tablespoons (30 ml)
maple syrup

1 teaspoon (5 ml) rose
water

Apple crumble is probably my all-time favorite dessert, and certainly one that evokes many childhood memories. I like to use several varieties, because some are sweeter, tarter, or crisper than others. Some keep their shape, while others break down under the crumble. Stick to one variety if you prefer, though. Walnuts lend a welcome buttery crunch to the crumble, and the rose-scented cream is a lovely, delicate accompaniment. Leaf lard is the fat from the kidneys and loin of the pig; you can substitute regular lard here. Soak and dehydrate the walnuts ahead of time to make them easier to digest (page 12).

Preheat the oven to 375°F (190°C, or gas mark 5). Place a flat baking sheet onto the middle shelf.

To make the crumble, pour the lemon juice in a large bowl. Cut the apples into quarters and each quarter into 3 wedges. As you cut them, toss the apple wedges in the lemon juice. Sprinkle over the cinnamon and 2 teaspoons of the coconut sugar, and mix well. Set aside.

Put the flours, salt, and lard in a separate bowl and rub together until it resembles coarse breadcrumbs. Wrap the walnuts in a clean tea towel, lightly crush them, and combine with the flour mixture with the remaining coconut sugar.

Transfer the apples to a 2½ (1,430 ml) pint ovenproof dish and lightly sprinkle over the topping. Place onto the hot baking sheet and bake for 45 minutes, or until the apples are bubbling. Turn the oven up to 400°F (200°C, or gas mark 6) for 10 minutes and continue cooking until the topping is crisp and golden.

To make the cream, put the coconut cream and maple syrup in a medium bowl and whip for 2 to 3 minutes until soft peaks form. Refrigerate while the crisp is in the oven. Just before serving, pour off any excess liquid and gently stir in the rose water.

Serve the crumble in bowls, each topped with a spoonful of rose-scented cream.

Walnuts	2
AIP COMPLIANT Omit walnuts.	
FREEZER-FRIENDLY Yes	
LOW FODMAP Choose low FODMAP fruits instead.	
COCONUT-FREE Sub honey for coconut sugar. Omit cream.	

CHERRY COFFEE CARDAMOM
SMOOTHIE

SERVES 2

PREP TIME:
5 MINUTES

1½ cups (232.5 g) frozen cherries

½ cup (125 ml) cold brew

¾ cup (185 ml) coconut milk

¼ cup (60 ml) cold chicken bone broth

⅛ teaspoon ground cardamom or seeds of 2 green cardamoms, crushed (Stage 1)

1 teaspoon (5 ml) vanilla extract

Pinch Himalayan pink salt

2 tablespoons (10 g) grass-fed collagen (optional)

4 ice cubes

This is a delicious way to get your daily coffee fix. Cherries, coffee, and cardamom are all rich sources of antioxidants, and coconut adds the healthy fat, which will keep you going until your next meal. This smoothie is also a different way to get in some gut-healing broth, or sneak it in undetected!

Put the cherries, cold brew, coconut milk, broth, cardamom, vanilla, salt, collagen (if using), and ice cubes in a blender. Blitz until smooth. Add more liquid if needed.

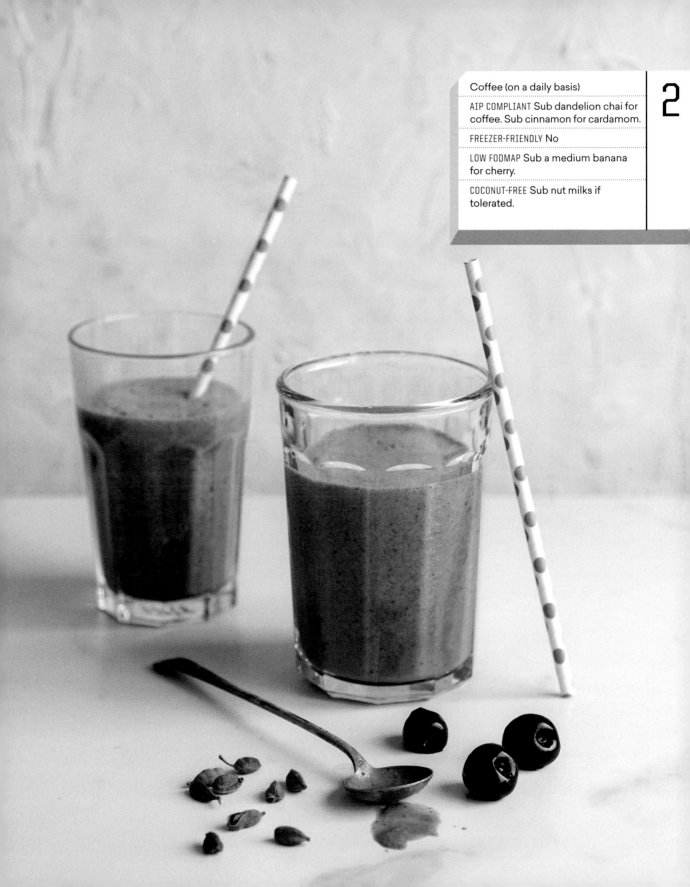

Coffee (on a daily basis)

AIP COMPLIANT Sub dandelion chai for coffee. Sub cinnamon for cardamom.

FREEZER-FRIENDLY No

LOW FODMAP Sub a medium banana for cherry.

COCONUT-FREE Sub nut milks if tolerated.

PAN-FRIED PINEAPPLE & BANANA
WITH MACADAMIA NUTS

SERVES 6

PREP TIME:
10 MINUTES,
PLUS SOAKING

COOK TIME:
10 MINUTES

2 tablespoons (28 g) ghee
(Stage 1) or butter (Stage 2)

2 teaspoons ground
cinnamon

½ small pineapple, cut into
6 wedges

3 small bananas, halved
lengthways

2 tablespoons (30 ml) maple
syrup

½ cup (67.5 g) macadamia
nuts, soaked, dehydrated,
and chopped

A few small fresh basil
leaves

Macadamia nuts add a buttery crunch to this dish that makes me think there's no better way to reintroduce them into your diet. They also have a much lower inflammatory omega-6 content than most nuts. Pan-frying brings out the flavor of pineapple, which is mellow and sublime. I love any excuse to snip some herbs into my food and basil is certainly a conversation starter. See page 12 for how to prepare the nuts for easier digestion.

Put a large frying pan over medium heat and add the ghee. Sprinkle over the cinnamon and add the pineapple. Leave for 2 minutes and then flip them over. As you do so, add the banana, cut sides down, and cook for 1 minute or so on either side. Drizzle over the maple syrup, turn the fruits to coat, and remove from the heat.

Divide the pineapple and banana between plates and spoon the buttery maple juices over the top. Sprinkle with macadamia nuts and 2 or 3 small basil leaves per person.

2

Macadamia nuts

AIP COMPLIANT Omit nuts. Sub extra
virgin olive oil.

FREEZER-FRIENDLY No

LOW FODMAP Choose green-tipped
bananas.

COCONUT-FREE Yes

BEET & ALMOND MILK
LATTE

SERVES 1

PREP TIME:
10 MINUTES

COOK TIME:
5 MINUTES

1 cup (250 ml) almond milk

1 teaspoon beet powder

¼–½ teaspoon ground ginger

¼–½ teaspoon ground cinnamon

Pinch Himalayan pink salt

Well worth the purchase, organic beet powder is available from many health stores or online. One teaspoon of beet powder is the equivalent of a whole fresh beet, and it can be added to smoothies, soups, and stews, as well as your Valentine's Day baking because it makes a good natural food dye. I've given you a couple of choices depending on the amount of spice you like.

Put the almond milk, beet powder, ginger, cinnamon, and salt in a small pan. Bring to a simmer, stirring. Finish with a milk frother if you have one, and pour into your favorite mug.

Almond milk	
AIP COMPLIANT Sub coconut milk.	2
FREEZER-FRIENDLY No	
LOW FODMAP No	
COCONUT-FREE Yes	

DANDELION CHAI

MAKES 2 CUPS
(500 ML)

PREP TIME:
15 MINUTES

COOK TIME:
10 MINUTES

1 cinnamon stick,
broken in two

1 star anise, broken
(Stage 1)

6 small black peppercorns,
lightly crushed (Stage 1)

3 whole cloves

1 teaspoon fennel seeds
(Stage 1)

4 green cardamom pods,
lightly crushed (Stage 1)

1-inch (2.5 cm) piece fresh
ginger, trimmed and sliced

1 dandelion root tea bag

Almond milk

Honey (optional)

Warming and spicy, this delicious caffeine-free hot beverage is also a useful digestive tonic and detoxifier. Dandelion root helps cleanse the liver and get the bile flowing, which is important since it digests fats and removes toxins from the body. If you haven't reintroduced any seed spices yet, I still highly recommend you sip a cup of plain dandelion root tea on a regular basis.

Put the spices in a pan together with 2 cups (500 ml) water and bring to a boil. Turn down the heat and simmer 4 minutes. Bring to a boil again and pour into a teapot. Add the dandelion root tea bag and infuse for 4 minutes.

Strain into two cups and add almond milk to taste, along with a little honey (if using).

2

Almond milk

AIP COMPLIANT Omit Stage 1 ingredients. Drink black or with coconut milk.

FREEZER-FRIENDLY No

LOW FODMAP No

COCONUT-FREE Yes

MULTI-VEGGIE KRAUT
WITH POPPY SEEDS

MAKES ONE 3-PINT
(1.5-LITER) JAR

PREP TIME:
15 MINUTES,
PLUS 30 MINUTES
STANDING

2 lb (900 g) white
cabbage, shredded

2 tablespoons (37.5 g)
sea salt

10 oz (280 g) carrots,
coarsely grated

14 oz (400 g) daikon,
coarsely grated

2 tablespoons (17.6 g)
poppy seeds

Sauerkraut is teaming with good bacteria, particularly lactobacillus, which is important to have in our gut microbiome. Lactobacillus helps to feed other good strains of bacteria and prevents pathogens from colonizing the gut. While this is a great combination of flavors, you can rotate the veggies and seeds or spices to keep it interesting. We like to eat some kind of probiotic food each day, and kraut is particularly delicious with the Hearty Veggie Bowl with Spice-Toasted Chickpeas (page 135) and Scromelette (page 90).

You will need an airtight 3-pint (1.5-liter) fermentation jar.

Put the cabbage in a large bowl and mix in the sea salt. Leave for 30 minutes for the salt to break down the cabbage, and then pound with closed fists for 5 minutes to release juices.

Add the carrots and daikon and continue pounding for 4 to 5 minutes. Mix in the poppy seeds and pack everything tightly into the jar. Push down as much as possible to submerge the vegetables in the juice and release any trapped air. Add glass weights or a tightly rolled cabbage leaf to ensure the kraut stays below the liquid, and prevent mold from growing.

Cover with a tea towel and leave on the countertop for 3 to 5 days. Store in the refrigerator.

RECIPE IMAGE APPEARS ON PAGE 40.

Poppy seeds	
AIP COMPLIANT	Omit poppy seeds.
FREEZER-FRIENDLY	No
LOW FODMAP	No
COCONUT-FREE	Yes

2

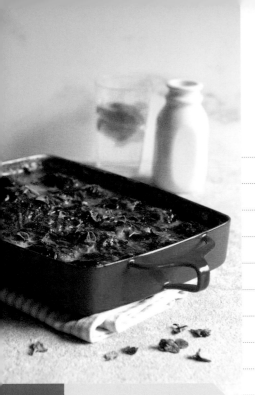

STAGE 3 RECIPES

RECIPE APPEARS ON PAGE 150.

reintroduction foods covered in this chapter

- bell peppers
- buttermilk
- cheese
- chickpeas
- cream cheese
- eggplant
- kefir
- lentils
- milk
- paprika
- potatoes (peeled)
- sour cream
- split peas
- whipping cream
- yogurt

CHAPTER FIVE

STAGE 3 RECIPES

YOUR SUCCESSFUL REINTRODUCTIONS in Stages 1 and 2 mean you have already done some gut healing—congratulations! We'll go a little cautiously in this stage, as this is where foods start to get a bit more challenging to reintroduce. You are ready for this, and I'm excited for you to try these new recipes.

If you're not reintroducing foods from the Stage 3 list (page 31) yet, that's no problem. The process is a lengthy one, so just settle into it and know that you are gifting your body the health it deserves. And keep in mind that the recipes are designed to be enjoyed as you make the appropriate modifications and substitutions—adapt them to what your body is ready for.

Some people do well with certain dairy foods and not others, because not all dairy is created equal when it comes to milk proteins. If you have celiac disease or gluten intolerance, you may find all dairy is a problem. And if you haven't been able to introduce ghee and butter into your diet, please enjoy the recipes in this chapter, but be sure to stay on the safe side and follow the AIP modifications.

If you can eat dairy, you're going to love the (very) Loaded Cheeseburger with Paprika Fries (page 153), Moussaka-Inspired Meatballs (page 150), and Pizza with Bocconcini, Anchovies, and Garden Vegetables (page 142). This stage also includes yogurt dressings, café-style beverages, and a range of desserts and baked treats to suit everyone and every occasion.

Chickpeas (garbanzo beans), lentils, and split peas are also Stage 3 reintroductions. (The remaining legumes should wait until you reach Stage 4.) These benefit the microbiome by adding essential fiber and increasing strains of bifidobacterium and lactobacillus species. Don't rush, though, and do prepare them properly to make them as digestible as possible (see page 13). Soaking dramatically decreases antinutrients, and is far less expensive than buying ready canned.

And don't forget to have a treat now and then. I cannot wait for you to try the Choco-Hazelnut Hummus (page 163). It's a heavenly treat for your microbiome and your taste buds!

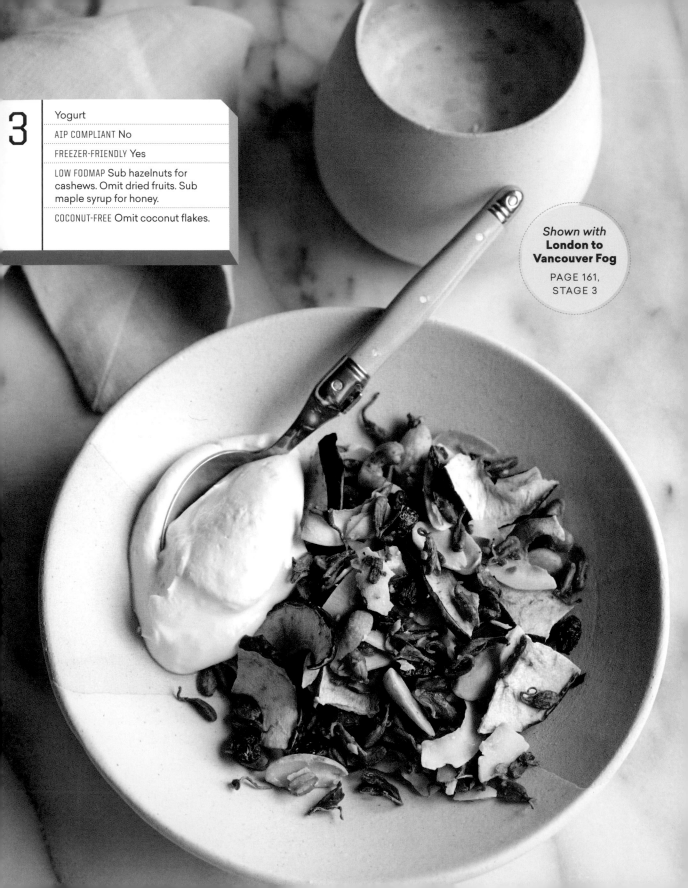

3 | Yogurt

AIP COMPLIANT No

FREEZER-FRIENDLY Yes

LOW FODMAP Sub hazelnuts for cashews. Omit dried fruits. Sub maple syrup for honey.

COCONUT-FREE Omit coconut flakes.

Shown with
London to Vancouver Fog
PAGE 161, STAGE 3

SPROUTED GRANOLA
WITH YOGURT

MAKES 7 CUPS

PREP TIME: 20 MINUTES, PLUS SOAKING/SPROUTING

DEHYDRATE TIME: 18 HOURS

GRANOLA

1 cup raw almonds, soaked overnight (Stage 2)

1 cup cashews, soaked for 6 hours (Stage 2)

1 cup sunflower seeds, soaked and sprouted (Stage 2)

1 cup pumpkin seeds, soaked and sprouted (Stage 2)

¼ cup coconut oil

¼ cup honey

1 cup toasted coconut flakes

½ cup raisins

½ teaspoon sea salt flakes

1½ cups bite-sized pieces dried apple

TO SERVE

½ cup yogurt per person

I came under a lot of pressure from the family to photograph this recipe quickly, because everyone wanted to dig in. It didn't disappoint! Start this recipe a few days in advance to allow the seeds to sprout. It makes them easier on the gut and increases nutrient levels that speed up healing. It is definitely worth the extra effort. If possible, use a dehydrator as the low temperature retains the life of the nuts and seeds.

To make the granola, squeeze the skins off the soaked almonds and split in half widthways. Dehydrate the nuts and seeds in thin layers at 105°F (41°C) overnight. Alternatively spread them out on two parchment-lined baking sheets and oven-dry at the lowest setting with the door left ajar for 6 hours. Check frequently and stir to ensure they are not burning. Once dried, remove and allow to cool.

Gently warm the coconut oil and honey in a small pan. Put the seeds, nuts, coconut flakes, and raisins in a large bowl and mix. Pour over the oil and honey, together with the salt, and mix again. Place back in the dehydrator set to 105°F (41°C). Leave for 4 hours.

Alternatively divide the mixture between parchment-lined baking sheets and put in the oven on the lowest setting for 20 minutes. Check frequently to make sure the granola doesn't burn.

Remove and transfer to large plates to cool. The mixture will harden as it cools. Mix in the dried apples.

To serve, put a cup of granola into a bowl and top with half a cup of yogurt. Store leftovers in an airtight container. Use within 3 weeks.

LENTIL PATTIES

MAKES 12

PREP TIME:
30 MINUTES, PLUS
SOAKING AND CHILLING

COOK TIME:
45 MINUTES

1 orange (¾ lb or 340 g) sweet potato, peeled and cut into ¾-inch (2 cm) cubes

1 white (¾ lb or 340 g) sweet potato, peeled and cut into ¾-inch (2 cm) cubes

1½ cups (288 g) sprouted green lentils

1 tablespoon (15 ml) extra virgin olive oil, plus more to fry

1 small leek, cut into quarters lengthways, and thinly sliced

Pinch Himalayan pink salt

½ teaspoon ground allspice (Stage 1)

½ teaspoon ground cumin (Stage 1)

¼ teaspoon ground turmeric

Pinch black pepper (Stage 1)

Zest of 1 large lime

¼ cup (15 g) chopped fresh flat-leaf parsley

2 tablespoons (12 g) chopped fresh mint

2 tablespoons (16.5 g) tapioca flour

Lime wedges

■■■■ Worth a spot at any meal, these delicious patties are particularly amazing for breakfast. Lentils are highly nutritious and have been shown to benefit the microbiome, which makes them a useful legume to reintroduce. Soaking and sprouting before cooking thoroughly minimizes antinutrients and maximizes nutrients, making lentils easier to digest. See page 13 for a how-to.

Steam the sweet potatoes for 12 minutes until soft. Drain, then mash until smooth and allow to cool.

At the same time, steam the lentils in another basket for 12 to 15 minutes. Cooking until soft makes them easier to digest. Transfer to a large plate and allow to cool.

Heat 1 tablespoon (15 ml) oil in a large frying pan and add the leeks. Cook gently for 6 minutes until softened. Stir in the salt and spices, and cook for 1 minute. Transfer to a large bowl and allow to cool.

Stir in the lime zest, parsley, and mint. Now add the sweet potatoes and lentils and mix well. Taste and adjust the seasoning if needed.

Line a baking sheet with parchment paper. Pack a ¼ cup measurement with the mixture and tap out onto your hand. Flatten slightly so the patty is roughly 2¾ inches (7 cm) in diameter. The mixture is quite loose at this stage but don't worry—it will firm up later. Dust with the tapioca flour and place on the baking sheet. Continue until you have 12 neat patties. Place the baking sheet in the fridge for 2 hours for the patties to firm up. Alternatively, you can pop them in the freezer for 20 minutes.

Put a large frying pan over medium heat and add a tablespoon (15 ml) of oil. Lightly dust the patties with tapioca flour once again.

Cook the patties in batches over medium heat for 2 to 3 minutes on one side; then turn them over and cook for 1 minute. They should be nicely browned and crispy on the outside.

Serve immediately, with the lime wedges. These patties are delicious with the Mint Mayonnaise on page 81.

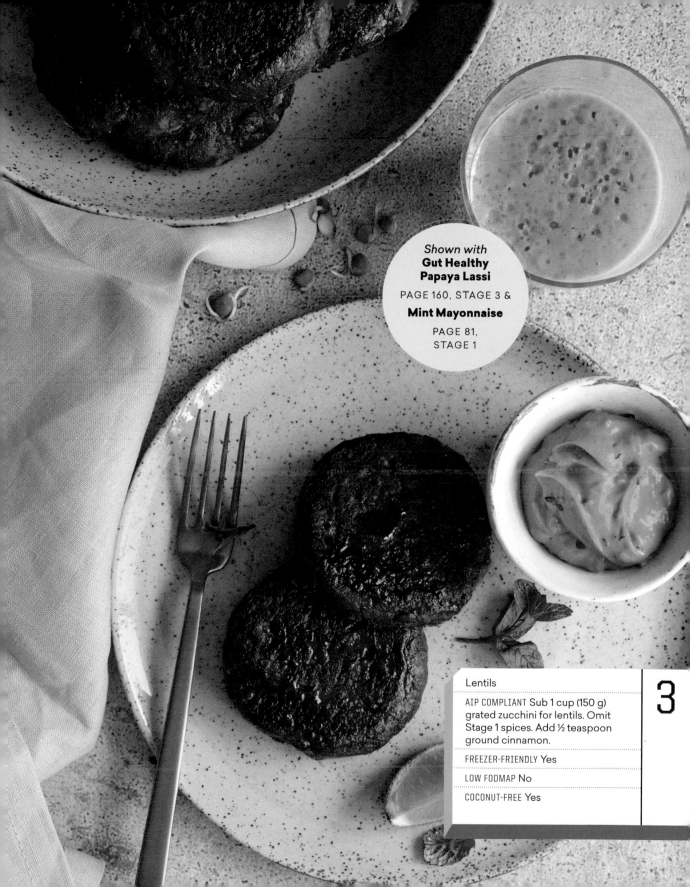

Shown with
**Gut Healthy
Papaya Lassi**
PAGE 160, STAGE 3 &
Mint Mayonnaise
PAGE 81,
STAGE 1

Lentils	3
AIP COMPLIANT Sub 1 cup (150 g) grated zucchini for lentils. Omit Stage 1 spices. Add ½ teaspoon ground cinnamon.	
FREEZER-FRIENDLY Yes	
LOW FODMAP No	
COCONUT-FREE Yes	

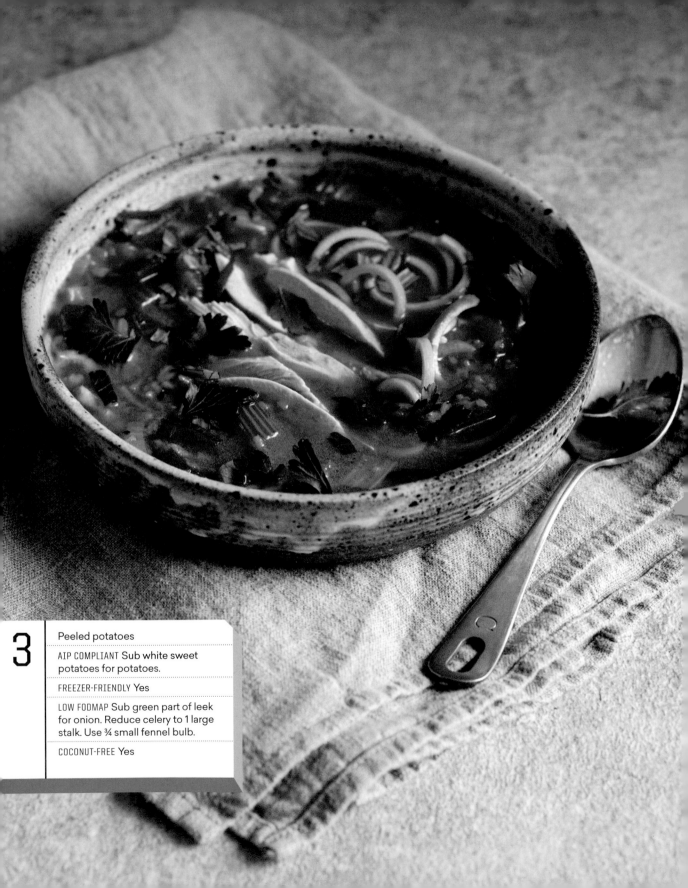

3

Peeled potatoes

AIP COMPLIANT Sub white sweet potatoes for potatoes.

FREEZER-FRIENDLY Yes

LOW FODMAP Sub green part of leek for onion. Reduce celery to 1 large stalk. Use ¾ small fennel bulb.

COCONUT-FREE Yes

CREAMY
CHICKEN NOODLE SOUP

SERVES 4

PREP TIME:
20 MINUTES

COOK TIME:
30 MINUTES

10 oz (280 g) white potato, peeled and finely grated

1 tablespoon (15 ml) extra virgin olive oil

1 medium onion, finely chopped

2 stalks celery, chopped

1 small fennel bulb, chopped, fronds reserved

2 large carrots, chopped

3 sprigs fresh thyme

1 large bay leaf

5 cups (1.3 L) chicken bone broth

Pinch sea salt

Pinch black pepper (Stage 1)

2-3 cups (450-675 g) shredded leftover chicken

2 tablespoons (8 g) chopped fresh tarragon

1 cup (60 g) chopped fresh flat-leaf parsley

2 medium zucchini, peeled and spiralized

▬▬▬ **This is just the thing for using up any roast chicken leftovers from the night before—or cook a couple of chicken joints just for this delicious soup. The grated potato breaks down into the soup for a thick and creamy texture. Zucchini noodles quickly fall apart when heated, so it's best to put them in the bowl rather than the pan.**

Put the potato in a large pan with ¾ cup (185 ml) water and cover. Cook 3 to 4 minutes over gentle heat, stirring occasionally.

Remove the lid, add the oil and onion, and cook for 5 minutes. Stir in the celery, fennel, and carrots.

Add the thyme, bay leaf, broth, salt, and pepper. Bring to a simmer, cover, and cook for 20 minutes, stirring occasionally to break down the potatoes.

When the veggies are tender, put the chicken in the pan and warm through. Remove from the heat, discard the bay leaf and add the herbs, including the reserved fennel fronds. Taste and adjust seasoning as desired.

Divide the zucchini noodles between bowls and pour over the soup. Wait for 4 to 5 minutes for the noodles to soften before serving.

SPLIT PEA SOUP
WITH SHRIMP & CASHEWS

SERVES 4

PREP TIME: 20 MINUTES, PLUS SOAKING

COOK TIME: 1¾ HOURS

3 tablespoons (45 ml) extra virgin olive oil, divided

1 medium yellow onion, chopped

2 large cloves garlic, minced

½ teaspoon ground turmeric

½ teaspoon ground ginger

1 teaspoon ground cumin (Stage 1)

2 cups (450 g) yellow split peas, soaked overnight

2 large carrots, grated

6 cups (1.5 L) chicken bone broth

1½ cups (45 g) chopped (½ bunch) spinach

Sea salt

Pinch black pepper (Stage 1)

½ cup (68 g) cashew nuts, soaked for 6 hours

16 large shrimp, peeled and deveined

2 scallions, cut in half and sliced lengthways into matchsticks

3

Split peas	
AIP COMPLIANT	No
FREEZER-FRIENDLY	Yes
LOW FODMAP	No
COCONUT-FREE	Yes

Split peas greatly benefit the microbiome by increasing the beneficial bacteria living there, particularly bifidobacterium and lactobacillus species. They are well worth a reintroduction attempt because they also have lower levels of lectins than other dried beans. This is a tasty, soothing soup that would also be wonderful made with soaked lentils. See page 13 for how to prepare split peas for cooking and improve their digestibility.

Heat 2 tablespoons (30 ml) oil in a large pan and add the onion. Cook gently for 6 to 8 minutes, or until softened, then add the garlic and spices. Cook for 1 to 2 minutes.

Drain and rinse the split peas and add to the pan, along with the grated carrots. Stir in the broth and bring to a simmer. Cover the pan and cook, stirring occasionally, for 1½ hours or until the peas have completely softened. Add the spinach and cook another 5 minutes until wilted. If you would like your soup silky smooth, transfer to a blender to purée. Do this carefully in batches (or, alternatively, use an immersion blender), adding more broth if needed. Season with salt and pepper to taste.

Meanwhile, rinse the cashews and dry with a clean kitchen towel. Put a frying pan over medium heat and add the nuts. Cook for 5 minutes, shaking from time to time so they don't burn. Remove from the frying pan and put on a plate to cool.

When the soup is ready, cook the shrimp. Heat a frying pan and add the remaining oil to the frying pan. Sprinkle the shrimp with a little salt and place in the hot pan. Leave for 2 to 3 minutes on one side until golden. Turn over and cook for 1 minute, or until cooked through.

Ladle the soup into bowls and garnish with the shrimp and scallions. Roughly chop the toasted cashews, scatter over the soup, and serve.

GRILLED GOAT CHEESE
WITH PAN-ROASTED GRAPES & SAGE

SERVES 2 AS
AN APPETIZER

PREP TIME:
10 MINUTES

COOK TIME:
10 MINUTES

1 tablespoon (15 ml) extra virgin olive oil

6-8 sage leaves

1 cup (150 g) red seedless grapes

2 tablespoons (30 ml) good-quality balsamic vinegar

1 small goat's Brie cheese with rind

Large handful baby salad leaves

Simple and absolutely delicious, this dish contains so many flavors. It's quite rich though, so you don't need very much. If you haven't introduced cheese, enjoy the basic principle with prosciutto or smoked salmon instead. So good!

Put a large sauté pan over medium heat and add the oil. Fry the sage leaves for 15 seconds, or until crisp. Remove and place on a paper towel.

Put the grapes in the pan and cook for 3 to 5 minutes, depending on their size, shaking the pan once in a while. Pour over the balsamic vinegar and bubble to a syrupy consistency.

At the same time, line a small baking sheet with parchment paper. Cut the goat cheese in half horizontally and put the two pieces onto the parchment, cut side up. Place under the broiler for 3 to 4 minutes until golden and bubbling.

Arrange the baby salad leaves on a platter and add the grapes and Brie. Drizzle over the balsamic glaze and top with the sage leaves.

Goat Brie cheese

AIP COMPLIANT Omit cheese and serve prosciutto.

FREEZER-FRIENDLY No

LOW FODMAP Balsamic vinegar is fine at 1 tablespoon (15 ml) per serving.

COCONUT-FREE Yes

3

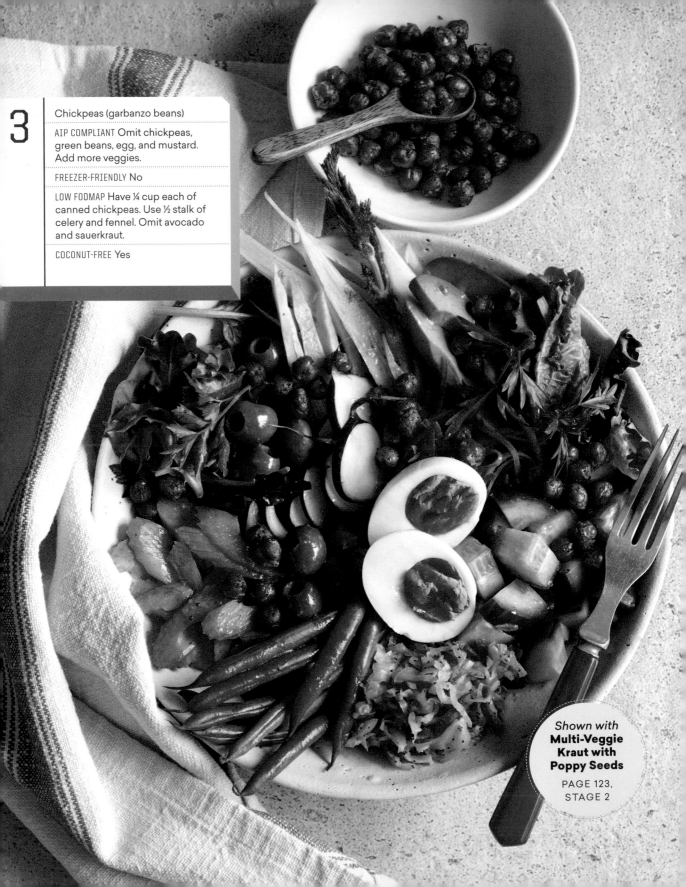

3 Chickpeas (garbanzo beans)

AIP COMPLIANT Omit chickpeas, green beans, egg, and mustard. Add more veggies.

FREEZER-FRIENDLY No

LOW FODMAP Have ¼ cup each of canned chickpeas. Use ½ stalk of celery and fennel. Omit avocado and sauerkraut.

COCONUT-FREE Yes

Shown with
Multi-Veggie Kraut with Poppy Seeds

PAGE 123, STAGE 2

HEARTY VEGGIE BOWL
WITH SPICE-TOASTED CHICKPEAS

SERVES 2

PREP TIME: 20 MINUTES

COOK TIME: 25 MINUTES

CHICKPEAS

1½ cups (15 oz can) cooked chickpeas, drained and rinsed

1 tablespoon (15 ml) extra virgin olive oil

¾ teaspoon kelp flakes

Pinch sea salt

SALAD

½ cucumber, chopped

4 radishes, thinly sliced

1 stalk celery, sliced on the diagonal

2 medium carrots, cut into thin ribbons

1 small fennel bulb, thinly sliced

Small handful green beans, tops trimmed, blanched (Stage 1)

Small handful baby greens

1 avocado, halved

½ cup (50 g) green olives

2 large spoonfuls Multi-Veggie Kraut (page 123)

DRESSING

1 teaspoon Windfall Country Mustard (Stage 1; page 79)

1 tablespoon (15 ml) lemon juice

3 tablespoons (45 ml) extra virgin olive oil

Pinch Himalayan pink salt

TO SERVE (OPTIONAL)

2 eggs, hard-boiled (Stage 2)

Spice-toasted chickpeas make a lovely snack or addition to salads. I like to use kelp flakes because they are so nutrient dense, but you could also use cumin (Stage 1), dried garlic, or flaked sea salt. See page 13 for how to prepare chickpeas from scratch.

Preheat the oven to 400°F (200°C, or gas mark 6).

To make the chickpeas, pat them dry and toss with the oil in a medium bowl. Spread out on a large rimmed baking sheet and bake for 20 minutes, shaking the baking sheet halfway through the baking time.

Remove the baking sheet and sprinkle the kelp flakes and salt over the chickpeas. Shake again to coat and return to the oven for 5 minutes.

Meanwhile, assemble the cucumber, radishes, celery, carrots, fennel, green beans, and baby greens in two large bowls. Add the toasted chickpeas and eggs (if using).

To make the dressing, whisk together the mustard, lemon juice, oil, and a pinch of salt. Pour the dressing over the salad, and serve.

TWICE BAKED SWEET POTATOES
WITH FETA

SERVES 4

PREP TIME:
15 MINUTES

COOK TIME:
70 MINUTES

4 medium sweet potatoes, scrubbed

1 tablespoon (15 ml) extra virgin olive oil

½ small red onion, chopped

¼ cup (24 g) chopped fresh mint

1 tablespoon (3 g) chopped fresh oregano

¼ cup (15 g) chopped fresh flat-leaf parsley

¼ cup (25 g) sliced black olives

1 tablespoon (8.6 g) capers, chopped

Pinch black pepper (Stage 1)

⅓ cup (50 g) crumbled feta cheese

Feta's slight acidity pairs beautifully with the sweetness of sweet potatoes. If you're starting to introduce feta, choose one made from sheep or goat milk; they contain less lactose than cow's milk. If you haven't reintroduced feta, sardines would work really well here and add a good boost of calcium and healthy fat.

Preheat oven to 400°F (200°C, or gas mark 6). Line a large baking sheet with parchment paper.

Make a slit down the center of each sweet potato but keep intact. Place on the baking sheet and cook 45 to 50 minutes until soft inside.

Meanwhile, put the oil in a small pan and add the red onion. Cook over gentle heat for 6 minutes, or until softened. Put in a medium bowl and allow to cool. Mix in the remaining ingredients apart from the feta and set aside.

When the sweet potatoes are cooked, scoop out the flesh and stir into the onion mixture. Divide into four equal portions and spoon back into the sweet potato shells. Sprinkle the feta over the top.

Return to the oven for 15 to 20 minutes until piping hot. Serve immediately.

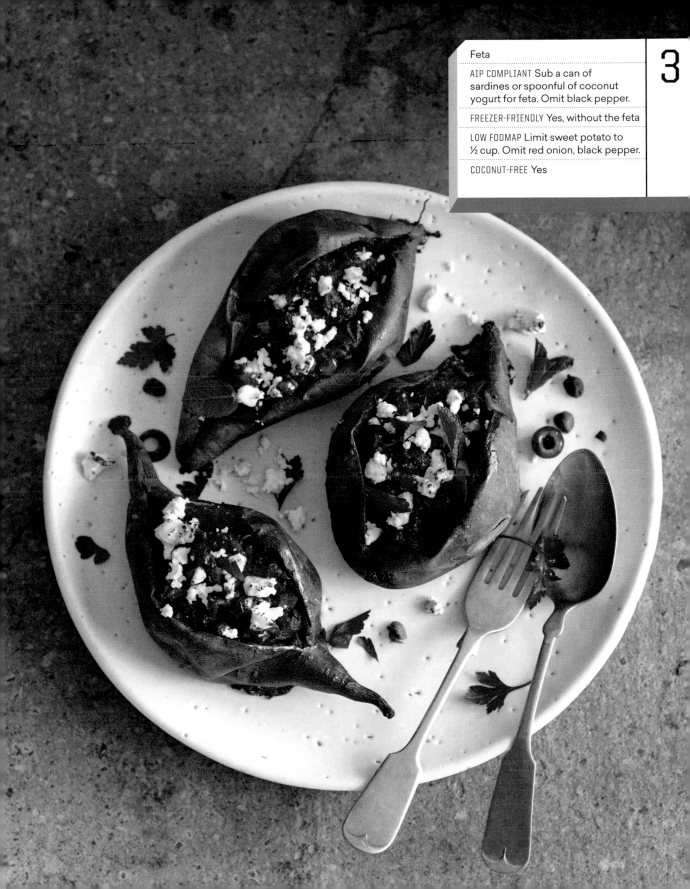

Feta

AIP COMPLIANT Sub a can of sardines or spoonful of coconut yogurt for feta. Omit black pepper.

FREEZER-FRIENDLY Yes, without the feta

LOW FODMAP Limit sweet potato to ½ cup. Omit red onion, black pepper.

COCONUT-FREE Yes

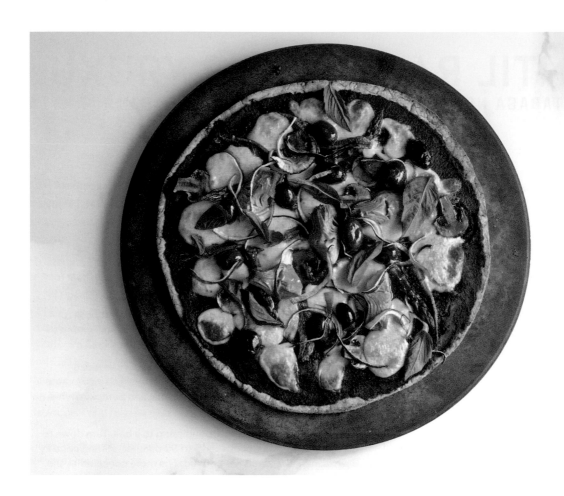

PIZZA
WITH BOCCONCINI, ANCHOVIES & GARDEN VEGETABLES

MAKES ONE 11-INCH
(28 CM) PIZZA, OR TWO
8-INCH (20 CM) PIZZAS

PREP TIME: 60 MINUTES,
PLUS 60 MINUTES TO
PROOF

COOK TIME: 60 MINUTES
FOR SAUCE, 30 MINUTES
FOR PIZZA

████████ Don't be put off by the inclusion of yeast in this recipe. It's not a deal breaker if you leave it out, but it does add the familiar taste and aroma that comes from traditional pizza dough. The "not-a-tomato" sauce makes enough for around 4 pizzas. If you're avoiding coconut, see your crust modifications on next page. Finally, you don't need to rely on cheese to make this pizza: A base sauce and a handful of favorite toppings will make you very happy.

BASE

1½ teaspoons dry active yeast

Pinch coconut sugar

¼ pint (150 ml) plus 2 tablespoons (30 ml) warm water, divided

1 cup (153 g) cassava flour

¼ cup (35 g) coconut flour

Pinch sea salt

2 tablespoons (30 ml) extra virgin olive oil

⅔ cup (81.6 g) warm mashed white sweet potato or ½ cup (122.5 g) pumpkin purée

"NOT-A-TOMATO" SAUCE (MAKES 3 CUPS [750 ML])

1 tablespoon (15 ml) extra virgin olive oil

1 small red onion, thinly sliced

4 cloves garlic, minced

2 tablespoons (30 ml) red wine vinegar

5 oz (140 g) red beet, grated

12 oz (340 g) golden beets, grated

8 oz (225 g) carrots, grated

¾ cup (183.7 g) pumpkin purée

1½ cups (375 g) chicken bone broth

Pinch sea salt

Pinch black pepper (Stage 1)

TOPPINGS (OPTIONAL)

½ container bocconcini or fresh mozzarella, torn

1 (2 oz or 55 g) can anchovies in salt, rinsed

4 asparagus spears, roughly chopped

4 artichoke hearts, quartered

⅓ cup (33.3 g) pitted mixed olives

8 button mushrooms, sliced

½ small red onion, thinly sliced

Extra virgin olive oil

Fresh basil leaves

To make the base, put the yeast and sugar in a small bowl and stir in 2 tablespoons (30 ml) warm water. Set aside for 5 to 10 minutes until the mixture is bubbly.

Put the flours and salt in a large bowl and make a well in the center. Pour in the remaining water, oil, sweet potato, and yeast mixture and bring together. Knead briefly on a lightly floured surface until you have a smooth, pillowy dough. Lightly grease the bowl and place the dough in the center. Cover with a tea towel and leave in a warm place for 1 hour.

Meanwhile, make the sauce. Heat the oil in a large pan. Add the onion and cook over gentle heat for 6 minutes, or until softened, then turn the heat up a little to get some color. Add the garlic and cook for 1 minute. Add the vinegar and, using a wooden spoon, deglaze the pan by scraping any sediment off the bottom.

Stir in the remaining sauce ingredients and bring to a simmer. Cover and cook for 40 minutes. Transfer to a blender and blend until smooth, adding more broth/water if needed. Set aside.

Place one or two pizza stones or flat baking sheets in the oven. Preheat to 450°F (230°C, or gas mark 8).

Place the dough on a 12-inch (30 cm) sheet of parchment and put another identical sheet on the top. Roll the dough into an 11-inch (28 cm) circle and tidy the edges. Alternatively, divide the dough into 2 even pieces and roll into 8-inch (20 cm) rounds. Cook for 12 minutes until firm.

Swirl spoonfuls of sauce over the top, followed by your choice of toppings. Cook for 10 to 15 minutes. Drizzle a little olive oil and scatter the basil leaves over top. Serve immediately.

NOTE: **Refrigerate leftover sauce in a sterilized jar for up to 2 weeks. For a coconut-free crust: Omit coconut flour and substitute an extra 2 tablespoons (19.5 g) cassava flour, ⅓ cup (45 g) tigernut flour, and 2 tablespoons (16.5 g) arrowroot.**

Mozzarella cheese	3
AIP COMPLIANT Omit mozzarella and add extra toppings.	
FREEZER-FRIENDLY Yes	
LOW FODMAP Crust is okay. Sauce is not. Avoid asparagus, artichoke, mushrooms, and onion.	
COCONUT-FREE See recipe in note above.	

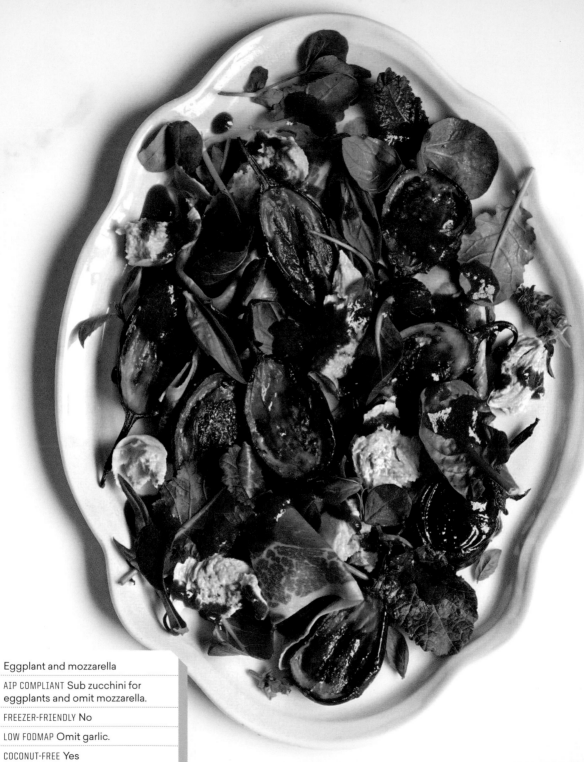

3   Eggplant and mozzarella

AIP COMPLIANT Sub zucchini for
eggplants and omit mozzarella.

FREEZER-FRIENDLY No

LOW FODMAP Omit garlic.

COCONUT-FREE Yes

BABY EGGPLANTS, PROSCIUTTO & MOZZARELLA
WITH BASIL DRESSING

SERVES 4

PREP TIME: 20 MINUTES

COOK TIME: 25 MINUTES

SALAD

2 tablespoons (30 ml) extra virgin olive oil

1 clove garlic, minced

Pinch sea salt

1 lb (12) baby eggplants, halved lengthways

12 slices prosciutto

1 mozzarella ball, torn into pieces

Large handful baby salad leaves

¼ cup (10 g) packed fresh basil

DRESSING

6 tablespoons (90 ml) extra virgin olive oil

1 tablespoon (15 ml) red wine vinegar

1 tablespoon (15 ml) lemon juice

1 clove garlic

½ cup (20 g) packed fresh basil

Pinch sea salt

If you can't get baby eggplants for this recipe, choose a couple of medium size and then brine and roast them in the way described in the Moussaka-Inspired Meatballs on page 150. Use this dressing with other salads or alongside roasted vegetables—it's so versatile.

Preheat the oven to 400°F (200°C, or gas mark 6).

To make the eggplants, put the oil, garlic, and salt in a large bowl. Add the eggplants and mix well to coat with the oil mixture.

Place cut side upward on a baking sheet and roast for 20 minutes until softened. Turn them over and cook for 5 minutes until golden brown. Remove and allow to cool.

Meanwhile, make the dressing. Put the oil, vinegar, lemon juice, garlic, basil, and salt in a blender. Blend until smooth. Taste and adjust the seasoning as needed.

Arrange the prosciutto, mozzarella, and salad leaves on a large serving platter. Add the eggplants and drizzle over the dressing.

Scatter the basil leaves over the salad and serve.

CHICKEN & CHICKPEA
MASALA

SERVES 4

PREP TIME: 20 MINUTES,
PLUS SOAKING

COOK TIME: 35 MINUTES

6-8 chicken thighs, skin on,
bone in

2 large shallots, peeled and
finely chopped

4 oz (110 g) brown
mushrooms, sliced

2 large cloves garlic,
minced

½ teaspoon ground
cinnamon

12 dried curry leaves

2 teaspoons dried
fenugreek (methi) leaves

½ teaspoon ground cumin
(Stage 1)

½ teaspoon ground
coriander (Stage 1)

Pinch black pepper
(Stage 1)

½ cup (122.5 g) pumpkin
purée

1 cup (250 ml) chicken
bone broth

1½ cups (360 g) cooked
chickpeas

Pinch sea salt

This one-pan meal makes me truly happy. Chicken thighs have so much flavor, and they are always succulent and tender. This recipe is complete with a serving of sautéed greens or salad, and the herbed cauli rice on page 100. See page 13 for how to prepare your chickpeas for this recipe.

Put a large sauté pan or frying pan over medium-high heat. Place the chicken thighs in the pan, skin side down, and brown them well. Remove and set aside, leaving the fat behind.

Turn the heat down to low and add the shallots and mushrooms. Cook for 3 minutes, or until softened, adding a little cooking fat if needed.

Add the garlic and spices and cook for 1 minute, stirring. Pour in a splash of water if the pan is starting to burn. Add the pumpkin and broth, bring back to the simmer, and add the chickpeas. Nestle the chicken thighs in the pan.

Cover and cook for 12 minutes, or until the chicken has cooked through. Remove the chicken and allow the remaining sauce to thicken slightly for 4 to 5 minutes. Add salt to taste and serve.

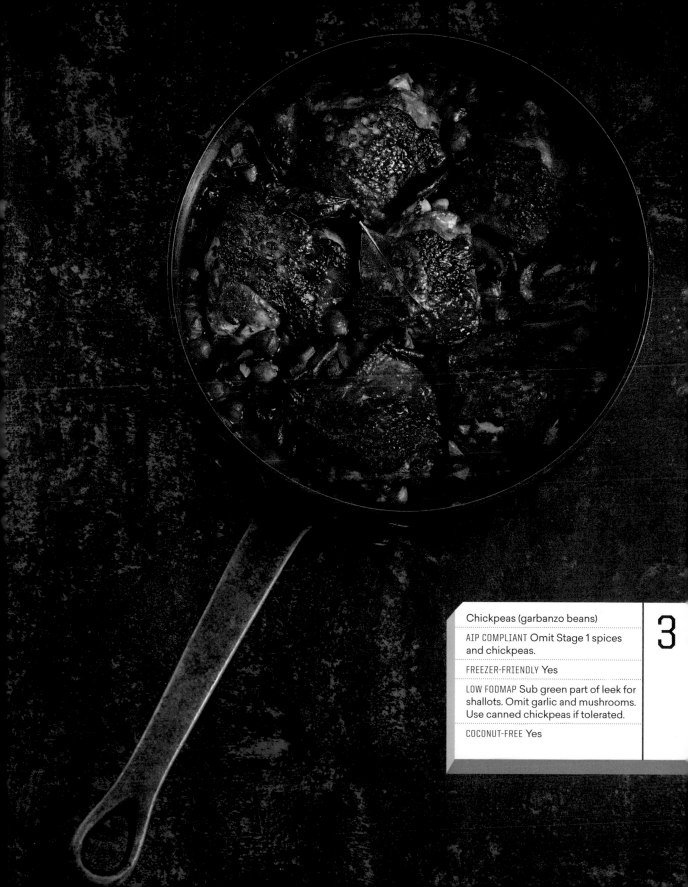

Chickpeas (garbanzo beans)

AIP COMPLIANT Omit Stage 1 spices and chickpeas.

FREEZER-FRIENDLY Yes

LOW FODMAP Sub green part of leek for shallots. Omit garlic and mushrooms. Use canned chickpeas if tolerated.

COCONUT-FREE Yes

3

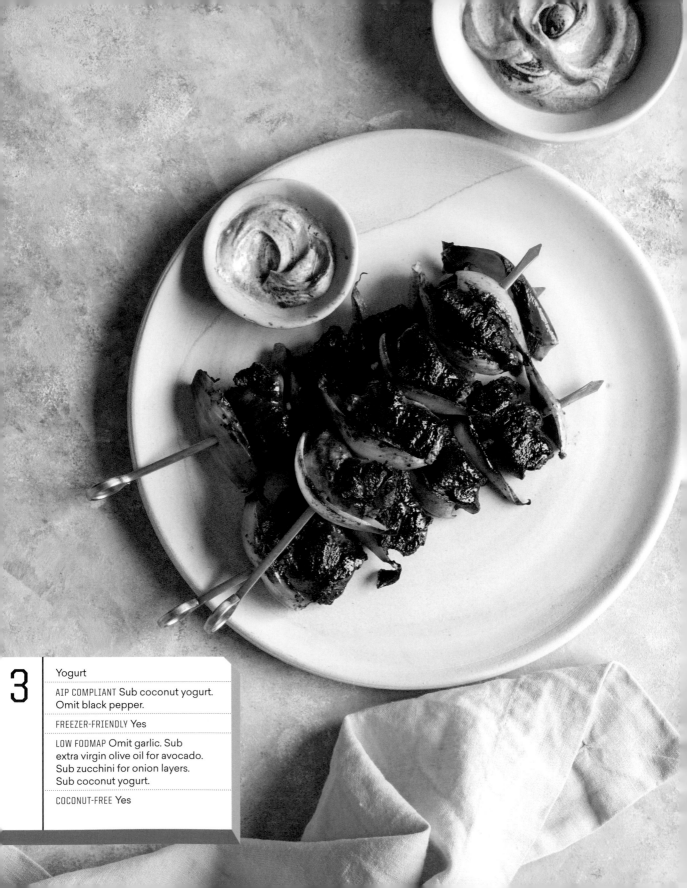

3

Yogurt

AIP COMPLIANT Sub coconut yogurt. Omit black pepper.

FREEZER-FRIENDLY Yes

LOW FODMAP Omit garlic. Sub extra virgin olive oil for avocado. Sub zucchini for onion layers. Sub coconut yogurt.

COCONUT-FREE Yes

MARINATED CHICKEN LIVER SKEWERS
OVER TURMERIC YOGURT

SERVES 4

PREP TIME: 35 MINUTES,
PLUS MARINATING

COOK TIME: 15 MINUTES

MARINADE

¼ cup (65 g) yogurt

3 tablespoons (45 ml)
avocado oil

2 cloves garlic, thinly sliced

¼ teaspoon ground
turmeric

½ teaspoon ground ginger

2 teaspoons (10 ml) lemon
juice

SKEWERS

7-8 slices bacon

¾ lb (340 g) chicken livers,
trimmed

1 small red onion, cut into
quarters and peeled into
layers

YOGURT

¼ teaspoon ground ginger

¼ teaspoon ground
turmeric

¼ cup (65 g) yogurt

½ teaspoon lemon juice

Pinch black pepper
(Stage 1)

Pinch sea salt

Whether you're a die-hard fan of organ meat or a little on the cautious side, you'll love eating this dish to ramp up your nutrition stores. Organ meat, particularly liver, is packed with the essential vitamins and minerals that will help the gut to heal, so please give it a try if you're on the fence. If you're still unconvinced, marinating before cooking will help to tenderize it. Plus you can never go wrong with bacon!

You will need 4 long metal or bamboo skewers. If using bamboo skewers, you will need to soak these for at last 30 minutes before cooking.

To make the marinade, place the yogurt, oil, garlic, turmeric, ginger, and lemon juice in a shallow dish and stir well. Add the chicken livers and combine well. Cover and set aside in a cool place for 1 hour.

To make the skewers, cut the bacon slices in half and wrap around each chicken liver. Push the skewer through a layer of onion followed by a wrapped chicken liver, threading through where the bacon joins. Continue alternating onions and chicken livers until all the livers are on the skewers. You should have around 4 bacon-wrapped livers on each one.

Put a griddle or frying pan over medium heat. When hot, lay the skewers over the top. Cook for 10 to 12 minutes, turning the skewers halfway through the cooking time and reducing the temperature to low so the bacon doesn't burn.

Meanwhile, make the yogurt dressing. Put ginger, turmeric, yogurt, lemon juice, and a pinch of pepper and salt in a small bowl. Mix together.

To serve, place a skewer on each plate and hand around the dressing at the table.

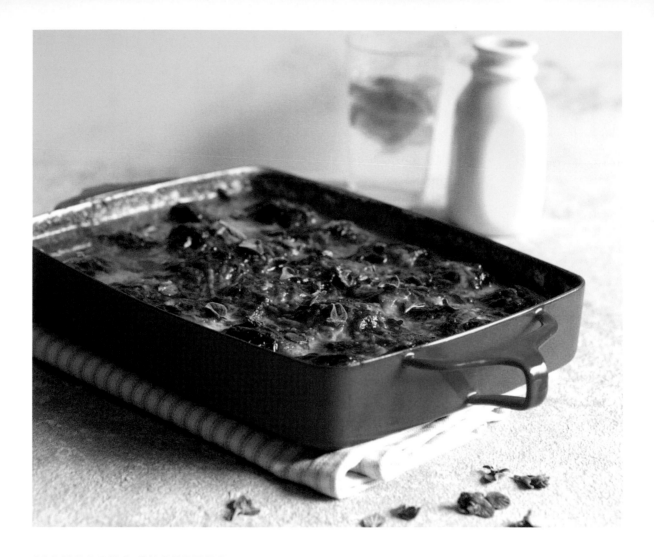

MOUSSAKA-INSPIRED
MEATBALLS

SERVES 4 TO 5

PREP TIME: 30 MINUTES,
PLUS BRINING

COOK TIME: 90 MINUTES

████ Instead of the traditional layers of meat and eggplant, I've incorporated them to form juicy meatballs. With a light covering of Mornay sauce over the top and a scattering of cheese, this might be your new family favorite. Pecorino is made with sheep's milk, which may be easier on the digestive system, but you could also use Parmesan (made from cow's milk) if you prefer.

MEATBALLS

2 tablespoons (36 g)
coarse sea salt

1 lb (450 g) eggplant,
cut lengthways into ½-inch
(1 cm) slices

3 tablespoons (45 ml) extra
virgin olive oil, divided

Pinch of sea salt

Pinch black or white
pepper (Stage 1)

1 large onion, finely
chopped

2 cloves garlic, minced

1½ teaspoons ground
cinnamon

1 tablespoon (2.4 g) fresh
thyme

2 tablespoons (8 g)
chopped fresh oregano

1¼ lb (560 g) ground beef
or lamb

MORNAY SAUCE

4 tablespoons (56 g) lard
or other solid fat

5 tablespoons (48.75 g)
cassava flour

1½ pints (860 ml) coconut
milk

Grating of fresh nutmeg
(Stage 1)

1 large bay leaf

1 cup (110 g) grated
pecorino, divided

Pinch sea salt

Pinch white pepper
(Stage 1)

Start by brining the eggplant. Put the coarse sea salt in a large bowl and add ½ cup (125 ml) boiled water. Stir to dissolve the salt and add 4 cups (1 L) cold water. Place the eggplant slices in the water, ensuring they are submerged, and leave for 30 minutes.

Preheat the oven to 400°F (200°C, or gas mark 6).

To make the meatballs, pat the eggplant dry. Brush each side of the eggplant slices with 1 tablespoon (15 ml) of the oil and sprinkle with salt and pepper. Place on a roasting tray and cook for 20 to 25 minutes, until the slices are light brown. Put the slices on a tray or a couple of large plates, and allow to cool.

Heat a large frying pan and add a tablespoon (15 ml) of oil, followed by the onion. Cook over low heat for 6 minutes, or until softened. Add the garlic and cinnamon, and cook for 1 minute. Transfer the mixture to a large plate, spreading it out so that it cools down quickly. Wipe out the frying pan with a paper towel. Reduce the oven temperature to 350°F (175°C, or gas mark 4).

Put the cooled eggplants in a food processor and blitz for 8 to 10 seconds to form a chunky paste. Add the sautéed onion mixture, together with the remaining meatball ingredients. Pulse until well combined. Using a medium ice cream/cookie scoop, form the mixture into 20 balls.

Put the frying pan back on the heat and add the remaining oil. Fry the meatballs for 6 minutes, or until browned all over.

At the same time, make the sauce. Melt the fat in a medium pan, add the cassava flour, and stir for 1 minute. Pour in the coconut milk, add the nutmeg and bay leaf, and stir continuously until boiling. Simmer for 3 minutes, stirring all the time to avoid any lumps forming. Reserve ⅓ cup of the cheese and add the remainder to the sauce. Remove the bay leaf and season with the salt, if needed, and the white pepper.

Arrange the meatballs in a 10 x 8–inch (26 x 20 cm) baking dish and pour over the sauce. Sprinkle the reserved cheese over the top and bake for 45 minutes, until golden brown and bubbling.

Eggplant and cheese

3

AIP COMPLIANT Sub zucchini for eggplant. Sub mace for nutmeg. Omit pepper. Sub ⅓ cup (25 g) nutritional yeast for cheese.

FREEZER-FRIENDLY Yes

LOW FODMAP Sub nutritional yeast for cheese. Sub green part of 2 leeks for onions. Omit garlic.

COCONUT-FREE Sub dairy milk if introduced. Or make white sauce from Luxury Fish Pie with Turmeric Mash (page 140)

BEEF STROGANOFF

SERVES 4

PREP TIME: 20 MINUTES

COOK TIME: 20 MINUTES

1 teaspoon (5 ml) extra virgin olive oil

1 lb (450 g) top sirloin steak, room temperature

Pinch sea salt

Pinch black pepper (Stage 1)

2 tablespoons (28 g) ghee (Stage 1) or butter (Stage 2)

1 medium onion, thinly sliced

8 oz (225 g) chestnut mushrooms, thinly sliced

Pinch ground allspice (Stage 1)

¾ cup (185 ml) beef bone broth

1 tablespoon (11 g) Windfall Country Mustard (Stage 1; page 79)

½ cup (115 g) sour cream

Slicing the steak before cooking makes it easy to overcook. For this comforting recipe I like to leave it whole, cook until rare, and leave it to rest while I make the sauce. Then, cut the steak into slices and warm them through in the sauce. If you find the slices a little too rare, you can continue cooking until they are how you like them!

Lightly coat both sides of the steak with the olive oil and season with salt and pepper. Put a large sauté pan over a high heat and add the steak. Sear for 2 minutes on either side until browned but still a little spongy when you press into the middle with a finger. The timing will depend on how thick they are. Remove and put on a warm plate.

Turn the heat down to low and add the ghee and onion. Cook gently for 3 minutes until almost softened, scraping up the color in the pan from the steak. Add the mushrooms, turn the heat to medium, and continue cooking for 3 to 4 minutes. Now add the allspice and cook for 1 minute.

Pour the broth into the pan and deglaze by scraping any sediment off the base.

Slice the steak into ¼-inch (6 mm) strips. Add to the pan together with the mustard and sour cream. Bring everything up to a simmer until the meat is hot. Taste and adjust the seasoning if needed.

Serve with mashed sweet potato or plain cauli rice (see page 100) to keep as AIP options. Alternatively, serve with mashed, peeled white potatoes (Stage 3) or white rice (Stage 4) if you have reintroduced them.

NOTE: **To make AIP compliant, sub lard or beef tallow for ghee. Sub 2 tablespoons (30 ml) coconut aminos for mustard. Sub mace for allspice. Add broth and reduce by half. Add ½ cup coconut cream (the solids remaining in a refrigerated can of coconut milk after the liquid is removed for other uses), and 1 teaspoon (5 ml) red wine vinegar and bring back to a simmer. Add the sliced meat to the pan and continue with the rest of the recipe.**

3

Sour cream
AIP COMPLIANT See note below
FREEZER-FRIENDLY Yes
LOW FODMAP No
COCONUT-FREE Yes

LOADED CHEESEBURGER
WITH PAPRIKA FRIES

SERVES 4
PREP TIME: 35 MINUTES
COOK TIME: 45 MINUTES

Everyone's favorite, this burger has a crunchy lettuce bun that's much healthier than the traditional bun. Choose a Swiss cheese or Cheddar as they contain less lactose than others and melt extremely well. Cook it all up and let everyone load up their own!

FRIES

2 large sweet potatoes, peeled and cut into ½-inch (1 cm) fries

1 tablespoon (8.25 g) tapioca flour

¾ teaspoon paprika

1 tablespoon (15 ml) avocado oil

Pinch sea salt

PATTIES

1 lb (450 g) grass-fed ground beef

Pinch sea salt

Pinch black pepper (Stage 1)

1-2 teaspoons (5-10 ml) avocado oil

TOPPINGS

2 tablespoons (30 ml) extra virgin olive oil, divided

1 large red onion, sliced thinly in rings

6 oz (170 g) brown mushrooms, sliced

4 slices bacon

1 large avocado, sliced

2-3 oz (55-85 g) Gruyère, Swiss, or Cheddar cheese, thinly sliced (optional Stage 3)

Nightshade-Free Brown Sauce (page 80)

Plain mayonnaise (Mint Mayonnaise minus the mint, page 81)

Multi-Veggie Kraut (page 123) or Kimchi (page 201)

1 medium iceberg lettuce, base trimmed

Preheat the oven to 425°F (220°C, or gas mark 7). Line two roasting trays with parchment paper.

To make the fries, toss the sweet potatoes, tapioca flour, and paprika in a bowl. Drizzle with oil and toss again. Spread the sweet potatoes over the trays, keeping space between them. Bake for 40 minutes, turning halfway. Remove from the oven and sprinkle with salt.

Meanwhile, make the burger patties. Divide and shape the ground beef into four, 4-inch (10 cm) patties. Season with salt and pepper. Set aside.

To make the toppings, heat 1 tablespoon (15 ml) of the oil in a large sauté pan and gently cook the onions for 6 minutes. Push them to one side of the pan and add the remaining oil and the mushrooms. Cook for 5 to 6 minutes. The onions should be caramelized and the mushrooms softened and browned.

Lay the bacon on a rimmed roasting tray and cook in the oven for 5 to 6 minutes. Remove and keep warm.

Place another large frying pan over medium-high heat and add the oil and patties. Fry for 5 to 6 minutes, turning halfway. Put a thin slice of cheese over each patty and let it melt.

Make a secret sauce with mayonnaise and brown sauce to taste.

Cut the lettuce into quarters and divide each in half. Lay down four chunks and remove enough layers to fit the patty. Spoon in the sauce, add a patty and load up your toppings. Top with more lettuce to form a bun. Serve the fries alongside.

Paprika and cheese

AIP COMPLIANT Omit paprika and cheese. Use plain ferments.

FREEZER-FRIENDLY Yes

LOW FODMAP Sub coconut oil for avocado. Omit onion, mushrooms, avocado, brown sauce, and ferments.

COCONUT-FREE Yes

3

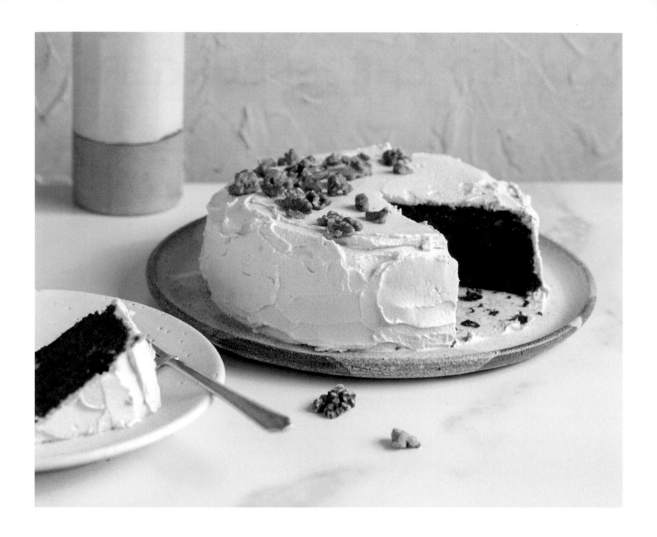

GARDEN CAKE
WITH CREAM CHEESE FROSTING

MAKES ONE 8-INCH
(20 CM) CAKE

PREP TIME:
40 MINUTES

COOK TIME:
60 MINUTES

Why stop at carrots? This is the cake equivalent of a vegetable patch, with almost 4 cups of veggies. Blackstrap molasses adds a hint of sweetness and packs a real punch in nutrients, especially calcium, iron, and magnesium. If you tolerate walnuts, add them for a bit of crunch. Soaking and dehydrating the walnuts will make them more easily digestible (page 12). If you have yet to reintroduce whole eggs, use 2 gelatin eggs instead (page 11).

CAKE

½ cup (125 ml) extra virgin olive oil

¾ cup (183.75 g) pumpkin purée

2 tablespoons (40 g) blackstrap molasses

1 tablespoon (15 ml) maple syrup

2 large eggs (Stage 2)

4 oz (110 g or 1 cup) grated carrots (2 medium)

6 oz (170 g or 1 cup) grated beets (1 medium)

6 oz (170 g or 1 packed cup) grated zucchini (1 small)

Zest of 1 large lemon

1¾ cup (195 g) tigernut flour

2 tablespoons (17.5 g) coconut flour

¼ cup (33 g) arrowroot starch

½ teaspoon ground cinnamon

⅛ teaspoon ground cloves

⅛ teaspoon ground mace

1½ teaspoons baking soda

Pinch sea salt

½ cup (60 g) walnut pieces, soaked, dried, and chopped (Stage 2)

FROSTING
(MAKES 2¼ CUPS
[ENOUGH FOR 1 CAKE])

1½ cups cream cheese (two 8 oz or 225 g packages), softened

1 cup (6 oz) butter, softened (Stage 2)

2 tablespoons (30 ml) maple syrup

2 teaspoons (10 ml) vanilla extract

Place a flat baking sheet in the oven and preheat to 350°F (175°C, or gas mark 4). Line an 8-inch (20 cm) baking tin with parchment paper.

To make the cake, put the oil, pumpkin purée, molasses, and maple syrup in your mixing bowl and beat to combine. If you are using eggs, add them one at a time, beating well between additions.

Add the carrots, beets, zucchini, and lemon zest and whisk briefly to incorporate. Tip in the flours, arrowroot, spices, baking soda, and sea salt, and mix again. If you are using gelatin eggs, see Kitchen Basics (page 11) for instructions and incorporate them here. Stir in the walnuts by hand.

Spoon the mixture into the prepared pan and place onto the pre-heated tray. Bake for 1 hour, or until the cake is firm and a skewer inserted into the center comes out clean.

Remove from the oven and allow to cool for about 15 minutes. Then turn out onto a wire rack to cool completely.

When the cake has cooled completely, make the frosting. Clean the bowl and paddle attachment. Beat the frosting ingredients on low speed for 1 minute, or until smooth, scraping down the sides when necessary.

Frost the cake once it has completely cooled, and serve.

Cream cheese

AIP COMPLIANT Omit the nuts from the cake. Omit frosting. Use 2 gelatin eggs.

FREEZER-FRIENDLY Yes

LOW FODMAP Sub carrots or zucchini for beets. Omit frosting.

COCONUT-FREE Sub tigernut flour for coconut.

3

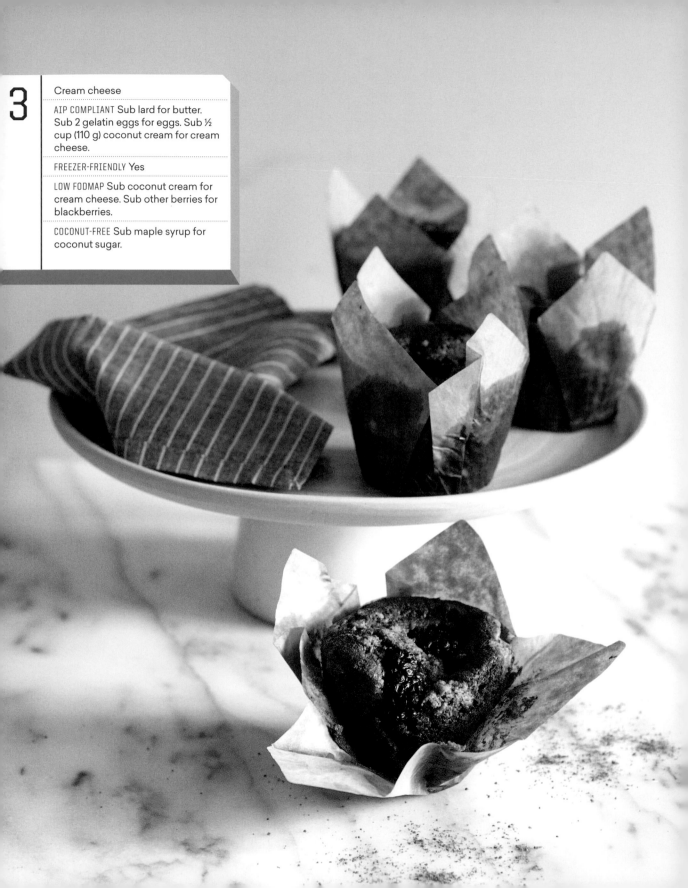

3 | Cream cheese

AIP COMPLIANT Sub lard for butter. Sub 2 gelatin eggs for eggs. Sub ½ cup (110 g) coconut cream for cream cheese.

FREEZER-FRIENDLY Yes

LOW FODMAP Sub coconut cream for cream cheese. Sub other berries for blackberries.

COCONUT-FREE Sub maple syrup for coconut sugar.

BLACKBERRY STREUSEL
MUFFINS

MAKES 8

PREP TIME:
30 MINUTES

COOK TIME:
20 MINUTES

Cream cheese paired with juicy berries make these muffins a more-ish treat. They're also great filled with coconut cream, so I like to keep a can of coconut milk in the refrigerator at all times for a constant supply. If you don't tolerate eggs, substitute two gelatin eggs instead (page 11).

STREUSEL TOPPING

⅓ cup (45 g) tigernut flour

¼ cup (56 g) butter (Stage 2)

¾ teaspoon ground cinnamon

Pinch sea salt

1 tablespoon (9 g) coconut sugar

MUFFINS

¼ cup (56 g) butter, softened (Stage 2)

¼ cup (60 ml) extra virgin olive oil

3 tablespoons (27 g) coconut sugar

2 eggs (Stage 2)

1 teaspoon (5 ml) vanilla extract

⅔ cup (154 g) cream cheese, softened

1¼ cups (140 g) tigernut flour

2 tablespoons (16.5 g) arrowroot starch

1½ teaspoons baking soda

Pinch sea salt

1 cup (6 oz or 170 g) blackberries

Preheat oven to 350°F (175°C, or gas mark 4). Line 8 cups of a 12-cup muffin tin.

To make the streusel topping, put the flour, butter, cinnamon, and a pinch of salt in a medium bowl and briefly rub between your fingers until the mixture resembles large crumbs. Stir in the sugar and sprinkle over 2 to 3 tablespoons (30 to 45 ml) cold water. Squeeze the mixture into small clumps and set aside in the fridge.

To make the muffins, put the butter, oil, and coconut sugar in the bowl of your stand mixer and beat until pale.

Beat in the eggs one at a time, followed by the vanilla. Once incorporated, turn the motor to a slow speed and mix in the cream cheese until just combined.

Add the flour, arrowroot, baking soda, and sea salt and combine again. If you are using gelatin eggs, see Kitchen Basics (page 11) for instructions and incorporate them here.

Spoon the mixture into the muffin cups and top with the blackberries. Divide the streusel mixture between the muffins and sprinkle lightly over the top.

Bake for 20 minutes, or until risen and firm around the edges. Leave in the tin for 10 minutes, before transferring to a wire rack to cool.

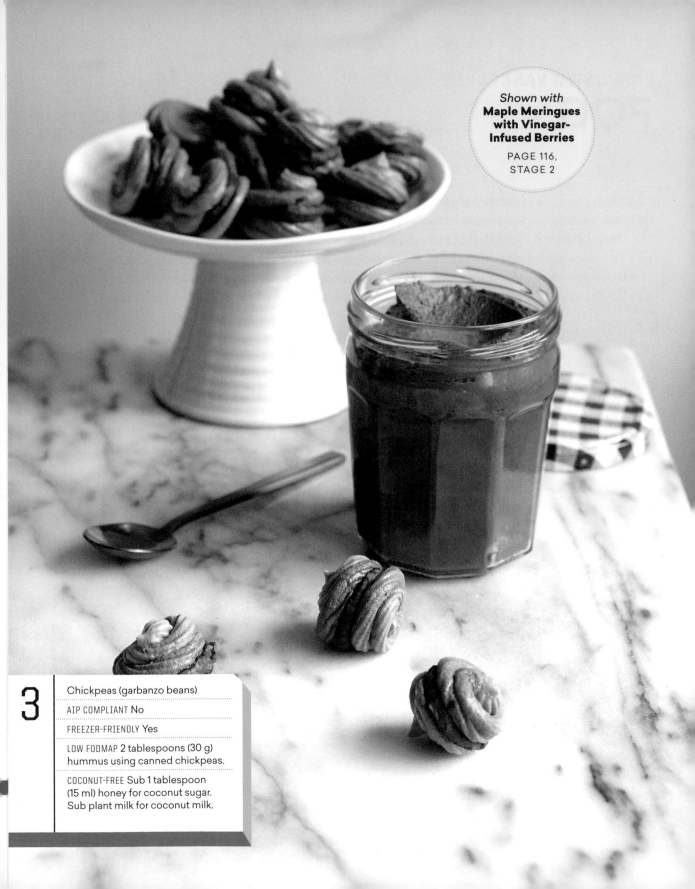

Shown with
Maple Meringues with Vinegar-Infused Berries

PAGE 116, STAGE 2

3	Chickpeas (garbanzo beans)
AIP COMPLIANT No
FREEZER-FRIENDLY Yes
LOW FODMAP 2 tablespoons (30 g) hummus using canned chickpeas.
COCONUT-FREE Sub 1 tablespoon (15 ml) honey for coconut sugar. Sub plant milk for coconut milk.

CHOCO-HAZELNUT
HUMMUS

MAKES 2 CUPS

PREP TIME:
15 MINUTES

1½ cups (360 g) cooked chickpeas

4 tablespoons (64 g) hazelnut butter (Stage 2)

2 tablespoons (30 ml) hazelnut oil (from the butter) (Stage 2) or extra virgin olive oil

4 tablespoons (22 g) cacao powder (Stage 1)

2 tablespoons (18 g) coconut sugar

Pinch sea salt

½ cup (125 ml) coconut milk

■■■■■ **Enjoy this winning treat on apple slices, spread between cakes and meringues, or as a dessert with slices of banana and yogurt. What can I say about this, other than you need it in your life! See page 13 for how to prepare the chickpeas for this recipe.**

Put the chickpeas, hazelnut butter, hazelnut oil, cacao powder, sugar, salt, and coconut milk in a food processor fitted with the small bowl. Blend until smooth and creamy.

Store in the refrigerator for up to 7 days.

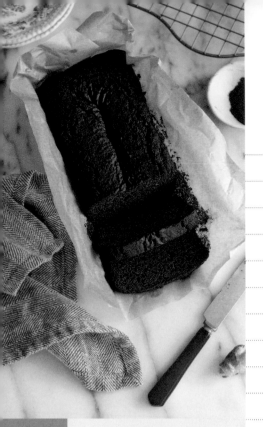

STAGE 4 RECIPES

reintroduction foods covered in this chapter

- alcohol (moderate)
- buckwheat
- cannellini beans
- cayenne pepper
- corn
- Great Northern beans
- hot peppers (chili)
- oats
- peanuts
- potatoes (unpeeled)
- rice
- tomatoes
- wild rice

RECIPE APPEARS ON PAGE 192.

CHAPTER SIX

STAGE 4 RECIPES

BEFORE YOU BEGIN this stage, let me encourage you to stop for a moment and recognize just how far you've come on your AIP journey. There may have been times when it felt like you were taking one step forward and two backward. You've come a long way. Your successes matter—well done!

This stage is a collection of the hardest foods to tolerate for people with compromised digestion and immune function. If you're not ready to reintroduce Stage 4 foods, don't worry. There's no rush! You can still enjoy plenty of easily adaptable recipes that will excite your taste buds.

Here's what to consider:

Before trying Stage 4 nightshades or their spices, make sure you've reintroduced some—if not all—of those listed in Stage 3 (page 31). The nightshade family can be especially hard for those with joint issues. I have to be cautious, so will have small portions on the odd occasion. Fish Tacos with Watermelon Tomato Salsa (page 180) and Gingerbread with a Hint of Cayenne (page 192) top my list. If you're having trouble with Stage 3 nightshades, concentrate on more healing first.

This stage also reintroduces gluten-free grains and pseudo-grains. I like the Lundberg brand for rice, which claims to have low levels of arsenic in their California-grown produce. Organic white basmati is my first choice—perfect in Childhood Chicken, Pineapple, and Rice (page 187), a favorite recipe for leftovers and pantry ingredients. Rice pudding is always welcome, especially when topped with blood oranges and saffron (page 195). Always buy organically grown corn. Otherwise there's a strong chance it's from a GMO crop. Oats, although naturally gluten-free, are subject to cross contamination; only buy from a company that manufactures oats that are certified gluten-free.

Stage 4 legumes (including peanuts) are harder to digest. Soaking is essential to break inhibitors down, followed by thorough cooking. Impress friends with Rosemary Slow-Cooked Lamb with Creamy Cannellini Mash (page 193) with caramelized onions.

A fermented food or drink with your meal helps aid digestion and populate the gut with healthy bacteria. I rotate sauerkraut (page 123), beet kvass (page 117), and kimchi (page 201). When homemade, the beneficial bacteria are often more varied than a probiotic supplement. They're also a reminder that eating to live is just as important as living to eat—something I truly hope you're experiencing in this book.

BUCKWHEAT TIGERNUT
PANCAKES

MAKES 10 TO 12

PREP TIME: 15 MINUTES

COOK TIME: 15 TO 20 MINUTES

½ cup (85 g) buckwheat flour

½ cup (55 g) tigernut flour

1 tablespoon (8.25 g) tapioca flour

1 teaspoon baking soda

Pinch sea salt

1 cup (250 ml) coconut milk

1 teaspoon (5 ml) raw apple cider vinegar

Avocado oil for frying

These are deliberately sweetener-free, so you can enjoy them with the Coffee Berry Compote (page 76) or with a little maple syrup drizzled over the top. Using sprouted buckwheat flour, which can be found online, will improve digestibility. If you're after an elimination-phase compliant version, see the note below.

Mix the flours, baking soda, and salt in a medium bowl and make a well in the center. Pour in the coconut milk and apple cider vinegar. Whisk to a smooth, thick batter.

Put a frying pan over medium heat and add a teaspoon of oil. When hot, drop in three ¼-cup measuring cups of the batter. Leave space in between and don't crowd the pan. Cook for 2 minutes, and then flip them for 1 to 2 minutes until cooked through. Add another teaspoon of oil and repeat the steps until all of the batter is cooked. You should get 10 to 12 pancakes.

NOTE: **For an AIP-friendly version, substitute these ingredients and follow the recipe directions:**
1 cup (110 g) tigernut flour
4 tablespoons tapioca flour
½ teaspoon ground cinnamon (optional)
½ teaspoon baking soda
Pinch sea salt
1 cup (250 ml) coconut milk
1 teaspoon (5 ml) raw apple cider vinegar

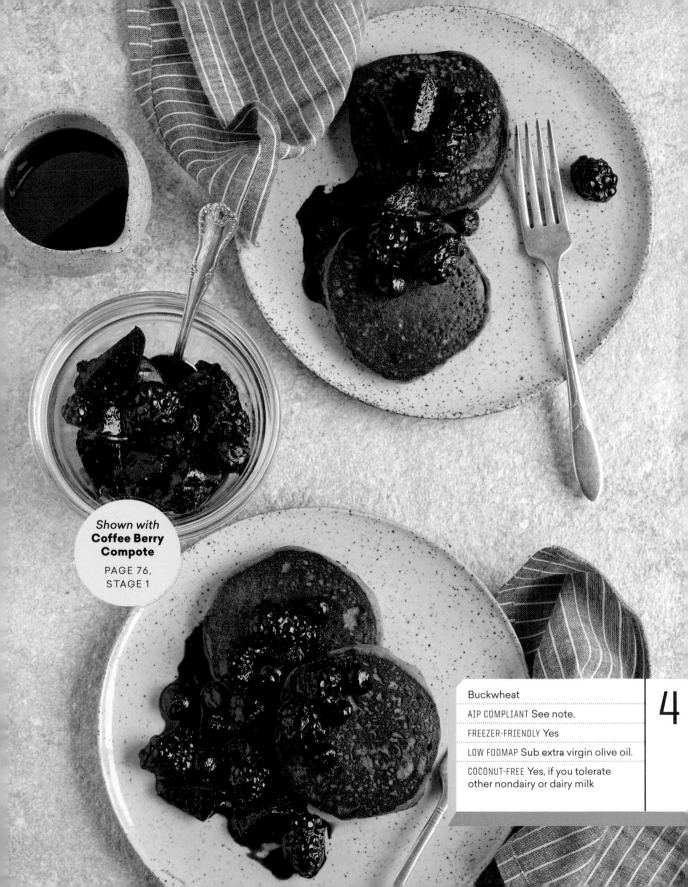

Shown with **Coffee Berry Compote** PAGE 76, STAGE 1

Buckwheat	4
AIP COMPLIANT See note.	
FREEZER-FRIENDLY Yes	
LOW FODMAP Sub extra virgin olive oil.	
COCONUT-FREE Yes, if you tolerate other nondairy or dairy milk	

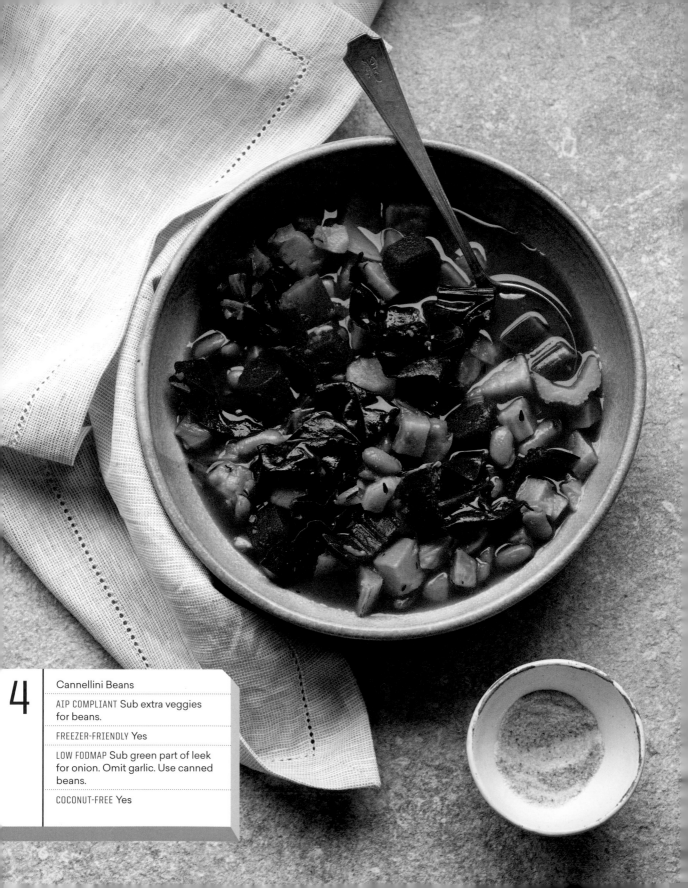

4

Cannellini Beans

AIP COMPLIANT Sub extra veggies for beans.

FREEZER-FRIENDLY Yes

LOW FODMAP Sub green part of leek for onion. Omit garlic. Use canned beans.

COCONUT-FREE Yes

CELERIAC, CHARD &
WHITE BEAN SOUP

SERVES 4

PREP TIME: 30 MINUTES,
PLUS SOAKING AND
PRECOOKING

COOK TIME: 55 MINUTES

2 tablespoons (28 g) lard
or other solid fat

1 large onion, chopped into
small dice

2 cloves garlic, minced

1 lb 3 oz (535 g) celeriac,
peeled and chopped into
¼-inch (6 mm) cubes

6 oz (170 g) carrots,
chopped into ½-inch (1 cm)
cubes

¾ lb (340 g) white sweet
potato, peeled and
chopped into ½-inch (1 cm)
cubes

3 sprigs fresh thyme

1 large bay leaf

3 cups (750 ml) chicken
bone broth

1½ cups (440 g, or 1 can)
cooked cannellini beans,
rinsed and drained

3 cups (165 g) packed
roughly chopped Swiss
chard (about 4 large
leaves)

Sea salt

Extra virgin olive oil

Celeriac, also known as celery root, is a funny-looking root vegetable that is a great source of vitamin K and calcium, both of which are essential nutrients for bone health. Rich in protein and fiber, cannellini beans make an excellent alternative to meat should you want a lighter meal. See page 11 for how to prepare them for this soup.

Put the fat in a large saucepan and add the onion. Cook over low heat for 6 minutes, or until softened. Add the garlic and cook for 1 minute.

Stir in the celeriac, carrots, sweet potato, thyme, and bay leaf, and put the lid on the pan. Cook over gentle heat for 20 minutes, or until just tender, stirring once in a while. The aim is to sweat the vegetables, rather than brown them, so add a tablespoon (15 ml) or two of water if needed.

Add the broth and beans. Bring to a simmer, put the lid back on, and cook for 15 minutes. Add the chard and simmer for 5 to 10 minutes until the vegetables have cooked through, and the chard has wilted.

Stir in salt to taste, and allow some of the beans to break down slightly and thicken the soup. Remove the thyme sprigs and bay leaf.

Ladle the soup into bowls and drizzle over a little olive oil.

MAPLE TURMERIC
OATS

SERVES 2

PREP TIME:
5 MINUTES,
PLUS SOAKING

COOK TIME:
10 TO 12 MINUTES

1 cup (156 g) certified
gluten-free steel-cut oats

1 tablespoon (15 ml)
lemon juice

2 tablespoons (28 g) ghee
(Stage 1) or coconut oil

2 tablespoons (30 ml)
maple syrup

½ teaspoon ground
turmeric

Pinch sea salt

Pinch black pepper
(Stage 1)

A great source of fiber, oats are known to lower cholesterol and increase levels of some strains of beneficial bacteria in the gut. Presoaking gives them a better flavor and creamier texture, and it speeds up cooking time. Purchase oats that are certified gluten-free because many brands are cross contaminated from wheat during processing. Steel-cut or rolled oats can't be home-sprouted; however, you can purchase them online. Add the black pepper if you tolerate it, because it improves the absorption of turmeric.

Put the oats in a bowl with the lemon juice and 2 cups (500 ml) filtered water. Cover and keep in the refrigerator for 24 hours.

When you are ready to eat, drain and rinse the oats well. Place them in a medium pan and add 2½ cups (625 ml) fresh filtered water. Bring to a simmer and cook for 10 to 12 minutes, or until the excess water has disappeared. Stir occasionally to prevent it from sticking to the bottom of the pan. Stir in the ghee.

Meanwhile, mix the maple syrup, turmeric, salt, and pepper together in a small bowl.

When the oatmeal is ready, turn off the heat and stir in the maple mixture. Pour into bowls and eat immediately.

4

Oats

AIP COMPLIANT No, but try the
No Oats Oatmeal (page 46).

FREEZER-FRIENDLY Yes

LOW FODMAP Yes

COCONUT-FREE Yes

CARROT, GINGER,
& WILD RICE SOUP

SERVES 8

PREP TIME: 30 MINUTES,
PLUS SOAKING

COOK TIME: 60 MINUTES

SOUP

1 tablespoon (15 ml) extra
virgin olive oil

1 large onion, thinly sliced

3 stalks celery, thinly sliced

2 lb (900 g) large carrots,
sliced into ½-inch (1 cm)
rounds

1 lb (450 g) celeriac (celery
root), cut into ¾-inch (2 cm)
cubes

1½ teaspoons freshly
grated ginger

Pinch sea salt

7 cups (1.8 liters) chicken
bone broth

RICE

⅔ cup (106.6 g) wild rice,
soaked overnight

1 tablespoon (15 ml) extra
virgin olive oil

4 stalks celery, cut in half
lengthways and thinly sliced

4 scallions, thinly sliced
on the diagonal

2 tablespoons (8 g) chopped
fresh tarragon

Zest of 1 lemon

Pinch sea salt

Wild rice, which is actually a wetland grass, is rich in protein, B vitamins, and many essential minerals. Rather than cooking the soup and rice together, I like to keep them separate. A mouthful of silky-smooth soup topped with the rice's nutty flavor and texture is deeply satisfying. See page 13 for how to prepare the rice.

To make the soup, heat the oil in a large pan and add the onion. Cook gently for 6 to 8 minutes until softened. Add the celery, carrots, celeriac, ginger, and a pinch of sea salt. Pour in the broth, cover, and cook for 50 minutes, or until the vegetables have softened. Carefully transfer to a blender, in batches, and blitz until smooth. Alternatively, you can use an immersion blender to purée the soup in the pan.

Meanwhile, prepare the rice. Rinse well and put in a medium pan with 3 cups (750 ml) water to cover. Bring to a boil, turn the heat down, and simmer for 30 minutes, or until the rice has split open and the ends are curling. While the rice is cooking, fill a kettle with water and bring to a boil. When ready, tip the rice into a sieve and pour over the boiling water. Drain well.

Put the oil in a medium frying pan and add the celery. Cook gently for 5 minutes, or until almost softened. Add the scallions and continue cooking 1 to 2 minutes, until softened but keeping their shape. Turn off the heat and stir in the rice, tarragon, lemon zest, and salt to taste.

Pour the soup into bowls and top with the rice mixture. Serve immediately.

Wild rice

AIP COMPLIANT Sub cauliflower rice
for the wild rice.

FREEZER-FRIENDLY Yes

LOW FODMAP Sub green part of 2
leeks for onion. Use green part of
scallions. Use 2 stalks celery total.

COCONUT-FREE Yes

4

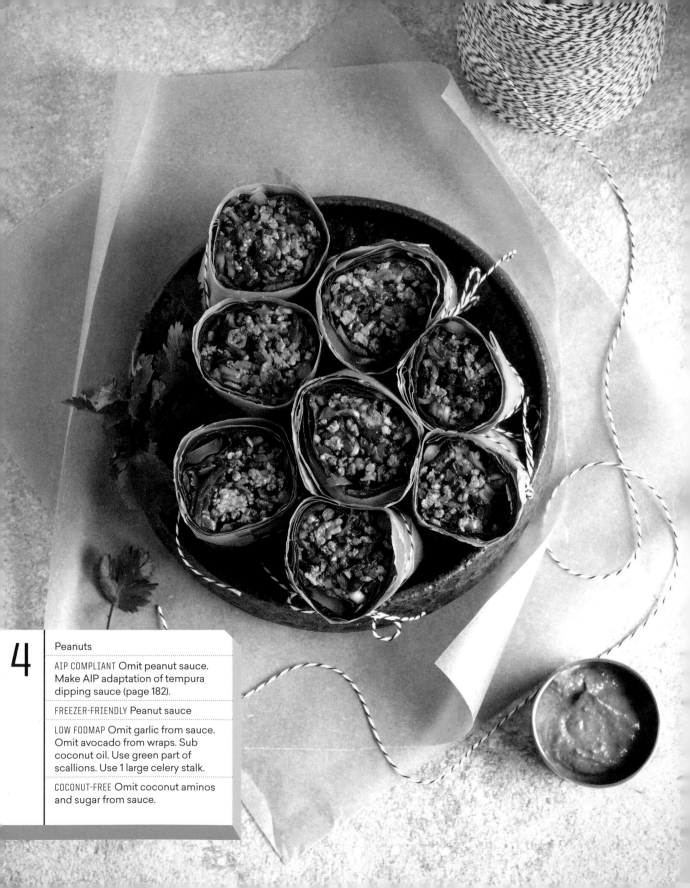

4

Peanuts

AIP COMPLIANT Omit peanut sauce. Make AIP adaptation of tempura dipping sauce (page 182).

FREEZER-FRIENDLY Peanut sauce

LOW FODMAP Omit garlic from sauce. Omit avocado from wraps. Sub coconut oil. Use green part of scallions. Use 1 large celery stalk.

COCONUT-FREE Omit coconut aminos and sugar from sauce.

COLLARD SALAD WRAPS
TO-GO WITH ROASTED PEANUT SAUCE

MAKES 4 FULL WRAPS
PLUS 1¾ CUPS (435 ML)
SAUCE

PREP TIME: 60 MINUTES,
PLUS SOAKING/DRYING

COOK TIME: 30 MINUTES

PEANUT SAUCE

1¾ cups (253.7 g) peanuts,
soaked and dehydrated

2 tablespoons (30 ml) coconut
aminos

2 tablespoons (30 ml) sesame oil

1 clove garlic, minced

1 teaspoon (5 ml) fish sauce

3 tablespoons (45 ml) lime juice

½ teaspoon coconut sugar

½ cup (125 ml) water

COLLARD WRAPS

1 tablespoon (15 ml) avocado oil

¾ lb (340 g) ground beef

2 tablespoons (30 ml) lime juice

2 tablespoons (30 ml) fish sauce

1 medium carrot, grated

2-inch (5 cm) piece daikon,
grated

2 stalks celery, thinly sliced

3 scallions, thinly sliced

½ cup (8 g) chopped fresh
cilantro

6–8 large collard green leaves

Soaking, drying, and oven roasting the peanuts may make this sauce seem like a labor of love. However, the recipe makes enough sauce for many wraps, and you could spoon the sauce over spiralized veggies or use it as a salad dressing. You can easily make the sauce with a different nut, such as almonds or cashews. See page 12 for how to soak and dehydrate nuts.

Preheat the oven to 350°F (175°C, or gas mark 4).

To make the peanut sauce, place the peanuts in the oven and roast for 15 to 20 minutes, shaking the baking sheet once in a while and frequently checking to prevent burning. Remove from the oven and set aside to cool.

Put the peanuts, coconut aminos, oil, garlic, lime juice, fish sauce, and sugar in a food processor. Blend for 4 minutes, or until you have smooth peanut butter. Slowly pour the water into the processor until you have a thick dipping consistency. Spoon into a jar.

Now prepare the collard wraps. Heat the oil over fairly high heat in a large frying pan and tip in the beef. Cook for 8 to 10 minutes until nearly crispy.

Pour in the fish sauce and lime juice, and cook until the liquid has evaporated. Tip into a large bowl to cool. Stir in the carrots, daikon, celery, scallions, and cilantro.

Meanwhile, bring a large pan of water to a boil. Fill a large bowl with ice water. With a sharp knife, shave off the protruding part of the collard stem but keep the whole leaf intact. Drop the collard leaves into the water and immediately turn off the heat. Leave for 30 seconds; then drain and transfer to the icy water to stop cooking further and to preserve the color. Once cooled, remove collards from the water, lay out on a paper towel–lined surface, and pat dry.

Put the beef mixture in the center of the leaves and roll up, burrito-style. Package each wrap with parchment paper and secure with kitchen string. Put the peanut sauce in a container and take with your collard wraps to-go!

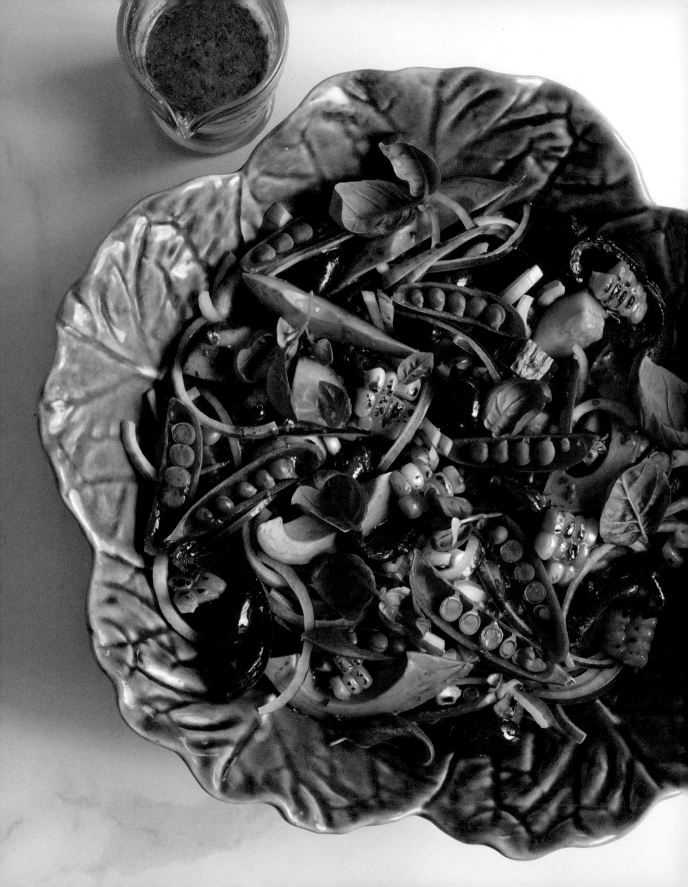

SUMMER SALAD
WITH HERBS & CHARRED CORN

SERVES 4
PREP TIME: 25 MINUTES
COOK TIME: 10 MINUTES

Although this recipe contains several reintroductions, it's super easy to adapt to whatever seasonal ingredient you have on hand and can tolerate. In fact, gather your favorite veggies, pour over the dressing, and you'll always have a great meal. This would also be amazing with the fish tacos (page 180). Be sure to use organic corn, because conventionally grown will likely be from GMO crops.

SALAD

1 ear of corn

1 teaspoon (5 ml) avocado or coconut oil

1 small red bell pepper, cut into thick slices (Stage 3)

1 small red onion, halved and thinly sliced

3 oz (85 g) sugar snap peas (Stage 1)

1 large avocado, sliced

½ English cucumber, quartered lengthways and chopped

½ cup (50 g) pitted black kalamata olives

½ cup (20 g) fresh basil leaves, torn if large

DRESSING

½ cup (8 g) fresh cilantro

5 tablespoons (75 ml) extra virgin olive oil

2 tablespoons (30 ml) white wine vinegar

1 tablespoon (15 ml) lime juice

Pinch sea salt

2 tablespoons (30 ml) whipping cream (Stage 3)

To make the salad, place the corn in a steamer basket and steam for 5 minutes. Remove and brush with avocado oil.

Place a griddle or grill pan over medium-high heat. Grill the corn for 5 minutes, turning occasionally until charred. Allow to slightly cool; then shave off the kernels and transfer to a large bowl. Grill the red pepper until lightly scorched.

Assemble all the salad ingredients in a large bowl.

To make the dressing, put the cilantro, oil, vinegar, lime juice, a pinch of salt, and the cream in a high-speed blender. Blend until smooth. Toss into the salad, and serve.

Corn

AIP COMPLIANT Sub other salad vegetables for corn and sugar snap peas. Sub coconut cream or water for cream, or omit.

FREEZER-FRIENDLY No

LOW FODMAP Sub green part of scallions for onion. Omit sugar snap peas and avocado. Sub coconut cream for cream, or omit. Avoid avocado oil.

COCONUT-FREE Yes

4

CRAB SALAD
WITH CUCUMBER RIBBONS & CHILI FLAKES

SERVES 2 AS AN
APPETIZER

PREP TIME: 15 MINUTES

SALAD

1 large ruby grapefruit,
peeled

1 long cucumber, peeled

4–5 oz (110–140 g) white
crabmeat

1 large avocado, sliced

1 tablespoon (6 g) chopped
fresh mint

Pinch chili flakes

DRESSING

2 tablespoons (30 ml) extra
virgin olive oil

Pinch ground ginger

Pinch sea salt

1 teaspoon (5 ml) white
wine vinegar

1 tablespoon (15 ml) juice
from the grapefruit

Salads don't get much more refreshing than this one. This is a lovely light meal for two—or two and a half if you have a cat that's as much a foodie as ours. If you can't get hold of fresh crabmeat, use large peeled and deveined shrimp instead. It'll still be delicious.

To prepare the grapefruit, segment it over a bowl, reserving the juice.

To make the dressing, whisk together the oil, ginger, salt, vinegar, and grapefruit juice. Taste and adjust the seasoning as needed.

To make the salad, use a sharp vegetable peeler to slice the cucumber into paper-thin ribbons and place in a bowl or on a serving platter. Add the grapefruit segments, crab, avocado, and mint. Pour over as much dressing as you like and sprinkle over the chili flakes. Serve immediately.

4

Chili flakes

AIP COMPLIANT Omit chili flakes.

FREEZER-FRIENDLY No

LOW FODMAP Omit avocado.

COCONUT-FREE Yes

LEMONY WHITE BEAN HUMMUS

SERVES 4

PREP TIME: 30 MINUTES

HUMMUS
(MAKES 4 CUPS
(900 G))

3 cups (546 g) cooked Great Northern beans

½ cup (120 g) tahini (Stage 2)

2 cloves garlic, minced

6-8 tablespoons (90-120 ml) lemon juice (Meyer, if possible)

½ cup (125 ml) extra virgin olive oil

Pinch sea salt

SALAD

6 cooked artichoke hearts, quartered

½ cucumber, thinly sliced

6 large radishes, thinly sliced

½ cup (50 g) pitted black Kalamata olives

½ cup (30 g) roughly chopped fresh flat-leaf parsley

Handful of arugula

¼ cup (10 g) fresh basil leaves

2 tablespoons (17.2 g) capers, rinsed and dried

Extra lemon juice

Extra virgin olive oil

This is a casual, everybody-dig-in sort of recipe that I like to make with Great Northern beans as the base for hummus. The mild, slightly nutty flavor works well here because rather than dominating the platter, it slips in quite nicely with all the different flavors. Of course, you can use chickpeas, the more traditional legume, if you prefer. See page 13 for how to prepare the beans for cooking.

To make the hummus, place the beans, tahini, garlic, lemon juice, oil, and a generous pinch of salt in a blender or food processor. Blend until very smooth. Taste and adjust seasoning as needed.

To make the salad, spread the hummus on a large serving platter. Arrange the artichoke, cucumber, radishes, olives, parsley, arugula, basil, and capers over the top. Squeeze over a little lemon juice, together with a drizzle of olive oil.

Serve with tortilla triangles (page 180), and allow everyone to help themselves.

Great Northern beans
AIP COMPLIANT Omit hummus.
FREEZER-FRIENDLY Hummus
LOW FODMAP Use canned beans. Omit garlic and artichokes. Enjoy ½ cup (110 g) hummus.
COCONUT-FREE Yes

4

SMASHED NEW POTATOES
WITH LEMON PESTO

SERVES 4 TO 5

PREP TIME:
20 MINUTES

COOK TIME:
40 MINUTES

POTATOES

1½ lb (675 g) new potatoes, washed but unpeeled

Pinch sea salt

2-3 tablespoons (30-45 ml) avocado or coconut oil

Grated Parmesan cheese (optional) (Stage 3)

PESTO

Zest of 1 lemon

2 tablespoons (30 ml) lemon juice

¼ cup chopped fresh chives

1 packed cup chopped fresh curly parsley

2 tablespoons chopped fresh tarragon

½ packed cup chopped fresh dill

1 clove garlic, minced

1 tablespoon capers, rinsed

½ cup (125 ml) extra virgin olive oil

▬▬▬ **There are so many ways to serve these potatoes—here's mine. You can also enjoy this recipe with sweet potatoes but, rather than boiling, I would cut them into new potato–size chunks and lightly steam before smashing and roasting. If you've reintroduced hard cheese already, feel free to grate some over.**

To make the potatoes, put them in a large pan of boiling salted water and simmer for 12 to 15 minutes until tender when pierced with a knife. Alternatively steam them. Drain and leave to cool for 5 minutes.

Preheat the oven to 425°F (220°C, or gas mark 7). Line 2 rimmed baking sheets with parchment paper.

Place the potatoes onto the baking sheets, leaving a gap between each one. Using a potato masher or back of a fork, press down on each potato to smash it to ½ inch (1 cm) in height. Drizzle over the oil and sprinkle with salt. Place the baking sheet in the oven and bake for 30 minutes, or until crispy and golden.

Meanwhile, make the pesto. Place the lemon zest and juice, chives, parsley, tarragon, dill, garlic, capers, and oil in a blender or food processor. Blitz until chunky.

Remove the potatoes from the oven and serve hot with the pesto and grated Parmesan.

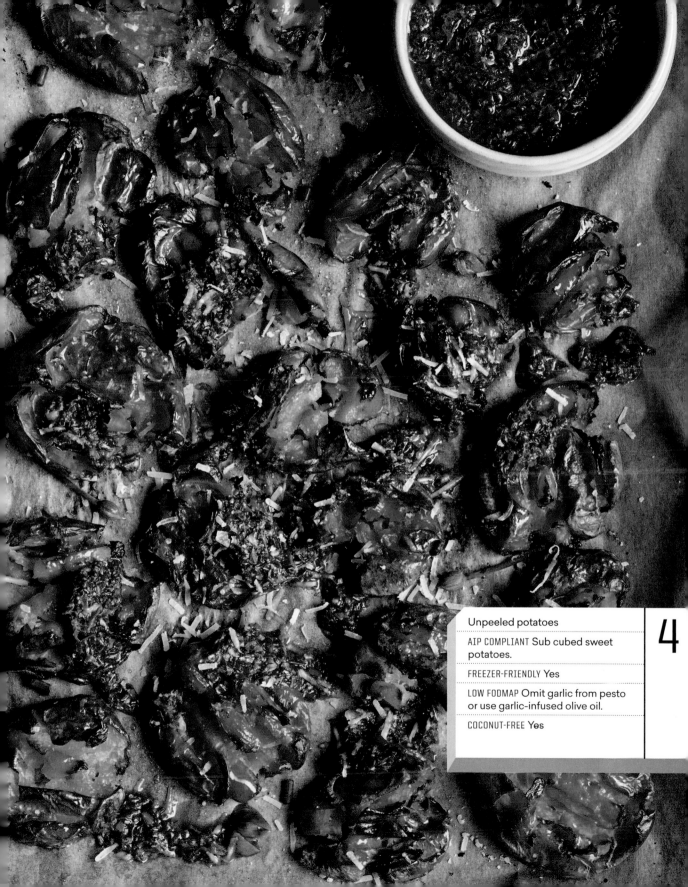

Unpeeled potatoes

AIP COMPLIANT Sub cubed sweet potatoes.

FREEZER-FRIENDLY Yes

LOW FODMAP Omit garlic from pesto or use garlic-infused olive oil.

COCONUT-FREE Yes

4

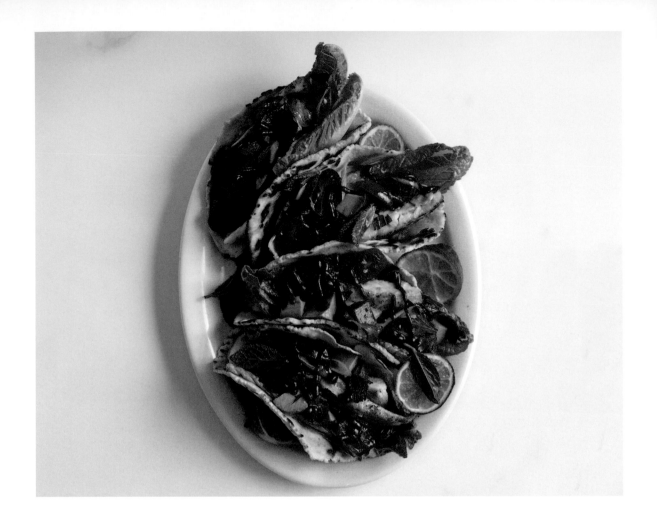

FISH TACOS
WITH WATERMELON TOMATO SALSA

SERVES 6

PREP TIME:
60 MINUTES

COOK TIME:
20 MINUTES

There's a lot going on in this recipe, but each part takes very little time, and the results are definitely worth it. Depending on how many tortillas you like to eat, you may want to double this part of the recipe. Even though cassava is surprisingly quite nutritious, I've increased the nutrients further by sneaking broth into my tortillas; you can use water if you prefer. If you have batches of Nightshade-Free Brown Sauce (page 80) or Mint Mayonnaise (page 81), you will want to get them out here.

TORTILLAS

1 cup and 1 tablespoon
(162 g) cassava flour

Pinch sea salt

¼ cup (60 ml) extra virgin
olive oil

⅔ cup (160 ml) cold chicken
bone broth

SALSA

½ small watermelon, rind
removed, cut into ½-inch
(1 cm) cubes

¾ cup (112.5 g) halved mixed
cherry tomatoes

1 avocado, cut into small
cubes

3 scallions, sliced on the
diagonal

¼ cup (4 g) chopped fresh
cilantro

¼ cup (24 g) chopped fresh
mint

DRESSING

5 tablespoons (75 ml) extra
virgin olive oil

1 tablespoon (15 ml) white
wine vinegar

4 tablespoons (60 ml) lime
juice

Pinch sea salt

FISH

2 tablespoons (19.5 g)
cassava flour

1 teaspoon garlic powder

Pinch sea salt

Zest of 1 large lime

4 fillets of firm skinless
white fish, such as cod,
tilapia, or halibut

1 tablespoon (15 ml) extra
virgin olive oil

To make the tortillas, put the flour and salt a large bowl. Pour in the oil and broth. Use a fork or your fingers to bring it together to form a dough. Knead for about 1 minute until you have a smooth dough. Roll into a log shape and slice into 6 even pieces. Roll each piece into a ball.

Cut 12 pieces of parchment paper into diameters of 7 inches (18 cm). If you have a tortilla press, lay one piece of parchment on the press, put a ball of dough in the center, and cover with a second piece of parchment. Press into a flat tortilla and set aside. Repeat with the remaining balls.

If you don't have a tortilla press, simply put each ball between two pieces of parchment paper and roll out to 6 inches (15 cm) in diameter.

To make the salsa, put all the salsa ingredients into a large serving bowl. Gently mix to combine.

To make the dressing, mix the ingredients in a small bowl. Pour over the salad and set aside to let the flavors infuse.

Now cook the tortillas. Put an empty heavy-based frying pan over medium heat. Place the first tortilla in the pan and cook for 1 minute. Turn it over and continue cooking for 1 minute. Place on a clean tea towel and loosely wrap. Repeat with all the tortillas, keeping them covered until they are all cooked.

Meanwhile, prepare the fish. Put the first four ingredients on a large plate and mix together. Press the fish fillets into the seasoned flour, coating well on both sides and dusting off the excess. Set aside.

When the tortillas are ready, add the olive oil to the pan. Fry the fish presentation side–down for 2 minutes, or until golden brown. Turn the fillets over and cook for 2 minutes, or until just cooked. The timing will depend on the thickness of your fillets.

To serve, place everything on plates or bowls and allow everyone to help themselves.

Tomatoes	4
AIP COMPLIANT Omit tomatoes.	
FREEZER-FRIENDLY Tortillas	
LOW FODMAP Omit avocado. Sub honeydew for watermelon. Use green part of scallions. Dust fish with tapioca flour, not garlic powder.	
COCONUT-FREE Yes	

SHRIMP & VEGETABLE
TEMPURA

SERVES 4

PREP TIME: 20 MINUTES

COOK TIME: 15 MINUTES

DIPPING SAUCE

2 tablespoons (30 ml) mandarin orange juice

3 tablespoons (45 ml) coconut aminos

1 tablespoon (15 ml) sesame oil (Stage 1)

1 tablespoon (15 ml) white wine vinegar

BATTER

¼ cup (39 g) cassava flour

¼ cup (33 g) tapioca flour

Pinch turmeric for color (optional)

Pinch sea salt

½ cup (125 ml) sparkling mineral water

AVOCADO OIL FOR FRYING

1 large firm avocado, peeled and cut into slices

4 radishes

8 baby corn

8 small heirloom carrots

8 thin asparagus spears

1 small delicata squash, sliced into half moons

12 large shrimp, peeled with tails left on

Tempura is a tasty way to increase your vegetable intake or encourage veggie-haters to eat up. You can use pretty much any vegetable, so don't feel you need to stick to my choice. Having said that, lightly battered avocado is pretty special. The blend of cassava and tapioca gives a light, crispy batter, which you could also use for onion rings. Have everything ready before starting this recipe, as it comes together quickly.

Line a large baking sheet or a couple of large plates with paper towels.

To make the dipping sauce, mix together the orange juice, coconut aminos, oil, and vinegar in a small bowl. Set aside.

To make the batter, put the flours, turmeric, and sea salt in a large bowl and make a well in the center. Pour in the sparkling water and whisk until smooth.

Put a medium pan over high heat and add a couple of inches of the avocado oil. It is ready when you drop in a little batter and it sizzles and rises to the top. Now turn the heat down to medium to avoid overheating.

Drop 2 or 3 veggie pieces into the batter and coat well. Using tongs or two forks, lift out and briefly shake over the bowl to remove any excess. Gently pop into the hot oil and cook for 1 minute, or until crispy and lightly golden. Transfer to the paper towels and keep warm until all batches are done.

When all the veggies are fried, repeat the process with the shrimp.

Transfer the tempura to a large platter and serve immediately, with the dipping sauce alongside.

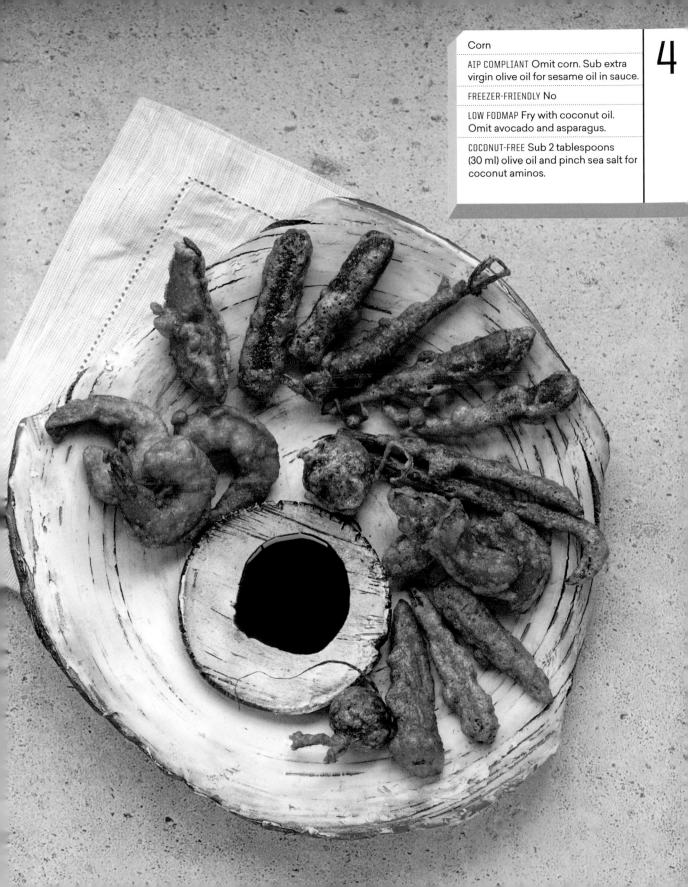

Corn

AIP COMPLIANT Omit corn. Sub extra virgin olive oil for sesame oil in sauce.

FREEZER-FRIENDLY No

LOW FODMAP Fry with coconut oil. Omit avocado and asparagus.

COCONUT-FREE Sub 2 tablespoons (30 ml) olive oil and pinch sea salt for coconut aminos.

CURRIED CHICKEN
& BUTTERNUT TRAY BAKE

SERVES 4

PREP TIME: 30 MINUTES

COOK TIME: 60 MINUTES

1 teaspoon ground cumin (Stage 1)

½ teaspoon ground coriander (Stage 1)

1 teaspoon ground turmeric

½ teaspoon ground cinnamon

½ teaspoon ground ginger

Pinch ground mace

¼ teaspoon chili powder

4 tablespoons (60 ml) extra virgin olive oil, divided

4 large chicken thighs, skin on, bone in

1 small butternut squash, cut into wedges

½ small cauliflower, cut into florets

2 small red onions, quartered

4 cloves garlic, whole and unpeeled

2 limes, halved

Pinch flaky sea salt

½ cup (8 g) chopped fresh cilantro

I love recipes that save on the washing up, and this one's no exception. It's an easily adaptable dish that will suit all your favorite veggies, so pack them in and get them tray baked.

Preheat oven to 400°F (200°C, or gas mark 6).

Mix the spices with 2 tablespoons (30 ml) of the oil in a small bowl, and coat the chicken thighs with the mixture. Set aside.

Arrange the chicken in a roasting pan with the squash, cauliflower, onions, and garlic. Lay the lime face down. Drizzle over the remaining oil and sprinkle with sea salt.

Roast for 45 to 50 minutes, turning the veggies halfway through the cooking time. Remove from the oven and scatter over the cilantro before serving.

4

Chili powder

AIP COMPLIANT Omit chili powder, cumin, and ground coriander.

FREEZER-FRIENDLY Yes

LOW FODMAP Sub kabocha squash for butternut. Sub small head of broccoli for cauli. Sub small fennel bulb for onions. Omit garlic.

COCONUT-FREE Yes

MUM'S WORK NIGHT
TUNA BAKE

SERVES 6

PREP TIME:
40 MINUTES

COOK TIME:
75 MINUTES

Another throwback to my childhood, and one more economical family meal that we always enjoyed—this tuna bake. Mum and I had great fun putting this recipe together recently, after several decades. Despite my changing it around somewhat, when I taste-tested it, I was suddenly sweet sixteen again!

TOPPING

5 slices bacon

⅓ cup (45 g) tigernut flour

1⅓ cup (5 oz or 140 g) coarsely riced cauliflower

SAUCE

4 tablespoons (59 g) lard or other solid fat

5 tablespoons (48.7 g) cassava flour

1½ pints (860 ml) coconut milk

1 large bay leaf

1 tablespoon (8.6 g) capers, chopped

2 cans (10 oz or 280 g) skipjack wild tuna

¾ cup (90 g) grated Cheddar cheese (Stage 3)

Pinch sea salt

Pinch white pepper (Stage 1)

BAKE

2 Roma tomatoes, thinly sliced

3 eggs, hard-boiled and sliced (Stage 2)

To make the topping, put the bacon slices on a baking sheet and broil in the oven for 8 to 10 minutes until crispy. Remove and transfer to a plate lined with paper towels and set aside. The bacon will harden as it cools.

Break up the bacon into small pieces with your hands and put in a medium bowl, together with the tigernut flour and riced cauliflower. Mix well and set aside.

Preheat the oven to 400°F (200°C, or gas mark 6).

To make the sauce, melt the fat in a medium pan, add the cassava flour, and stir for 1 minute. Pour in the coconut milk, add the bay leaf, and stir continuously until boiling. Simmer for 3 minutes, stirring, to avoid any lumps forming. Remove the bay leaf and stir in the capers, tuna, and cheese. Taste and season with the salt if needed, and white pepper, if using.

To assemble the bake, pour half the tuna sauce into 2½-pint (1.4-liter) oven-proof dish. Layer the tomatoes over the mixture, followed by the egg slices. Pour over the remainder of the tuna mixture.

Finally, lightly sprinkle over the bacon topping. Place on a baking sheet and pop in the oven for 45 to 50 minutes until bubbling and browned on the top.

Tomatoes	
AIP COMPLIANT Sub sautéed mushrooms and leeks for tomatoes. Sub ⅓ cup (25 g) nutritional yeast for Cheddar. Omit egg.	
FREEZER-FRIENDLY Yes	
LOW FODMAP Mix bacon and ¼ cup (30 g) Cheddar cheese for topping.	
COCONUT-FREE Yes, if reintroduced other milks.	

4

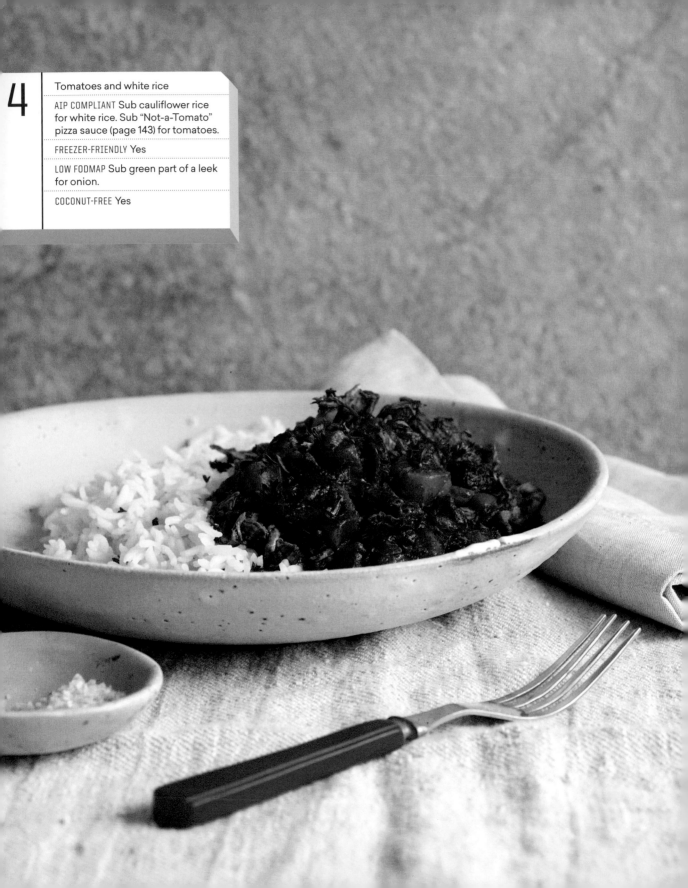

4 Tomatoes and white rice

AIP COMPLIANT Sub cauliflower rice for white rice. Sub "Not-a-Tomato" pizza sauce (page 143) for tomatoes.

FREEZER-FRIENDLY Yes

LOW FODMAP Sub green part of a leek for onion.

COCONUT-FREE Yes

CHILDHOOD
CHICKEN, PINEAPPLE, & RICE

SERVES 2 TO 3

PREP TIME:
15 MINUTES

COOK TIME:
25 MINUTES

1 tablespoon (15 ml) extra virgin olive oil

1 medium onion, chopped

1 cup (½ of 14.5 oz can) diced tomatoes

1 cup (250 ml) chicken bone broth

Pinch sea salt

Pinch black pepper (Stage 1)

6 oz (170 g) pineapple, cut into ½-inch (1 cm) chunks

6 oz (170 g) leftover chicken, shredded

⅓ cup (20 g) chopped fresh curly parsley

Cooked white basmati rice (see Resources on page 202)

Welcome to my childhood! Here's a throwback to when my brother and I would beg Mum to make this. It was really a way of using up roast chicken from the night before with a few added bits and pieces she'd find in the cupboard. The original also contained a small can of sweetcorn—you can add it if you like. White rice is known to contain differing levels of arsenic. See page 13 for how to prepare it.

Heat a large pan and add the oil and onion. Sauté over gentle heat for 6 minutes, or until softened.

Add the tomatoes, broth, and a pinch of sea salt and black pepper. Bring to a simmer and cook for 12 minutes, or until the liquid has reduced by half.

Next add the pineapple and chicken and cook for a few minutes more until hot, pouring in a little more broth or water, if needed. Taste and adjust the seasoning if you like.

Toss with the parsley and serve on cooked rice.

VIETNAMESE PORK
WITH NOODLES & ROASTED PEANUTS

SERVES 4

PREP TIME: 35 MINUTES, PLUS
SOAKING/DEHYDRATING

COOK TIME: 20 MINUTES

3 tablespoons (27 g) raw
peanuts, soaked and dehydrated

2 teaspoons (10 ml) avocado oil

1 lb (450 g) pork tenderloin, thinly
sliced

4 cloves garlic, thinly sliced

2-inch (5 cm) piece ginger, thinly
sliced

2 lemongrass stalks, thinly sliced

3 cups (750 ml) chicken bone
broth

2 tablespoons (30 ml) fish sauce

4 tablespoons (60 ml) coconut
aminos

Juice of ½ lime (2 tablespoons
or 30 ml)

8 oz (225 g) packet dried rice
noodles

2 cups beansprouts (Stage 1)

3½-inch (8.5 cm) piece daikon,
cut into matchsticks

2 medium carrots, cut into 4-inch
(10 cm) matchsticks

3 scallions, cut lengthways into
4-inch (10 cm) strips

¼ cup (24 g) fresh mint

¾ cup (30 g) fresh Thai or regular
basil leaves

1 cup (16 g) fresh cilantro

1 lime, cut into wedges

Vietnamese cuisine is among the healthiest in the world because it's usually very fresh and cooked quickly. The bulk of time spent is in the preparation, but once that's done, your meal comes together in no time. This particular recipe is half soup, half stir-fry. Soaking and dehydrating the peanuts before roasting will make them more digestible (see page 12).

Heat a wok or large sauté pan over medium heat and lightly toast the peanuts for a couple of minutes or so. Remove and set aside.

To make the pork, add the oil and pork to the pan and stir-fry for 4 minutes, or until cooked through. Transfer to a warm plate.

Add more oil to the sauté pan if needed, followed by the garlic, ginger, and lemongrass. Cook for a minute or two, being careful not to let them burn. Pour in the broth, fish sauce, coconut aminos, and lime juice and bring to a simmer. Cook for 5 to 6 minutes to infuse the broth.

Meanwhile, cook the noodles in a large pan of boiling water, according to the manufacturer's instructions.

Divide the broth, pork, and noodles between the bowls. Place the garnishes on a large plate and the peanuts in a small bowl. Allow everyone to help themselves.

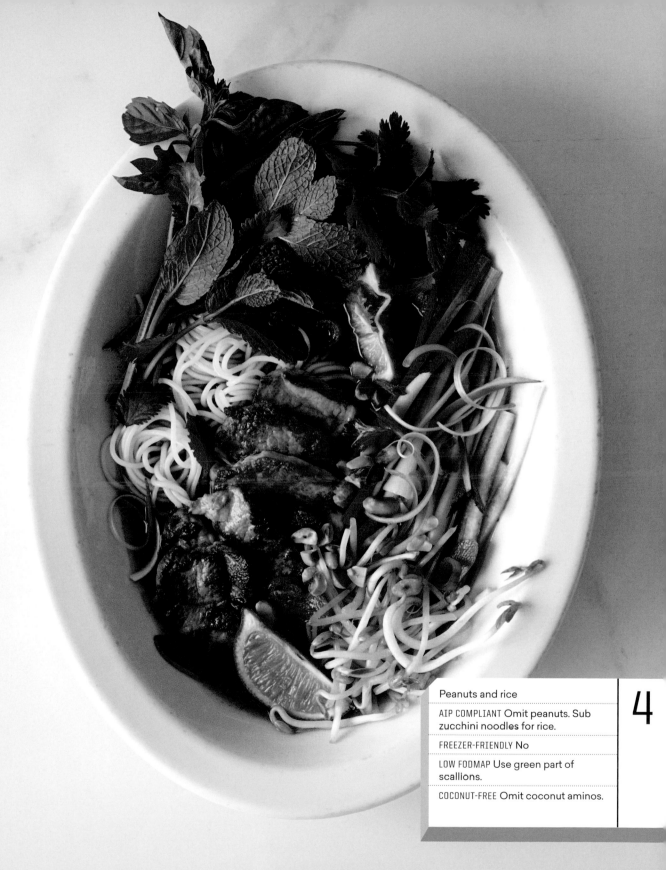

Peanuts and rice

AIP COMPLIANT Omit peanuts. Sub zucchini noodles for rice.

FREEZER-FRIENDLY No

LOW FODMAP Use green part of scallions.

COCONUT-FREE Omit coconut aminos.

4

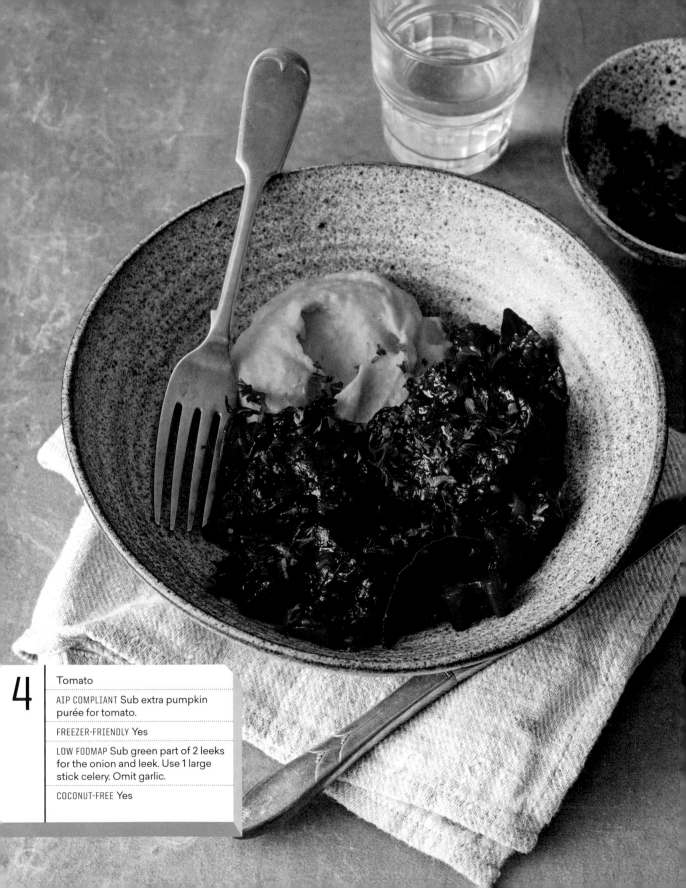

4

Tomato

AIP COMPLIANT Sub extra pumpkin purée for tomato.

FREEZER-FRIENDLY Yes

LOW FODMAP Sub green part of 2 leeks for the onion and leek. Use 1 large stick celery. Omit garlic.

COCONUT-FREE Yes

OXTAIL STEW

SERVES 4

PREP TIME:
30 MINUTES

COOK TIME:
3½ HOURS

1 tablespoon (15 ml)
extra virgin olive oil

3 lb (1.4 kg) oxtail cut into
1½-inch (3.5 cm) chunks

1 large red onion, chopped

1 large leek, sliced

3 large sticks celery,
chopped

2 carrots, chopped

2 cloves garlic, minced

2 bay leaves

4 sprigs fresh thyme

¼ cup (60 ml) red wine
vinegar

¼ cup (61.25 g) pumpkin
purée

2 tablespoons (32 g)
tomato paste

Pinch Himalayan pink salt

2½ cups (652 ml) beef
bone broth

½ cup (30 g) chopped fresh
flat-leaf parsley

Oxtail is one of my favorite ways to eat beef. It is also a rich source of gelatin and collagen, which is necessary for gut strengthening and repair. Oxtail needs to be cooked low and slow until the meat lifts away from the bone, but it's worth the wait because the end result is the most intense flavor that practically melts in your mouth. Get your butcher to chop the oxtail into chunks for you.

Preheat the oven to 300°F (150°C, or gas mark 2).

Place the oil in a large Dutch oven over medium-high heat and brown the oxtail in batches.

Remove from the pan, turn the temperature down to low, and add the vegetables, garlic, bay leaves, and thyme. Cook for 5 to 6 minutes, or until the onions have softened.

Turn the heat back up to medium and pour in the vinegar, pumpkin purée, and tomato paste. Cook for a couple of minutes, scraping the bottom of the pan to release the sediment and add flavor.

Return the oxtail and juices back to the pan, nestle them under the vegetables, and pour over the broth. Bring to a simmer, cover, and put in the oven.

Cook for 3 hours, until the meat is falling off the bone. Sprinkle with parsley and serve.

CHERRY CACAO NIB
OAT COOKIES

MAKES 16
JUMBO COOKIES

PREP TIME:
15 MINUTES

COOK TIME:
12 MINUTES

½ cup (60 g) dried cherries

4 cups (624 g) certified gluten-free rolled oats, divided

½ teaspoon baking soda

Pinch sea salt

½ cup (125 ml) melted coconut oil

½ cup (125 ml) honey

2 tablespoons (18 g) coconut sugar

½ cup (120 g) tahini (or other seed/nut butter) (Stage 2)

2 large eggs and an egg yolk (Stage 2)

2 teaspoons (10 ml) vanilla extract

4 tablespoons (43.75 g) cacao nibs (Stage 1)

■■■■ I've never been much of a cookie fan, but now I'm wondering how I've gone through life without these! Be sure to purchase certified gluten-free oats, and look for cherries that have been dried without seed oils or sweetener. If you can't find them, substitute large, juicy unadulterated raisins instead. While these cookies are a toothsome jumbo size, you could easily make 28 to 30 modest ones, adjusting the cooking time accordingly!

Start by plumping the dried cherries. Put them in a small bowl, pour over enough boiling water to cover, and leave for 20 minutes. Drain and place on a paper towel until cool.

Preheat the oven to 350°F (175°C, or gas mark 4). Line three baking sheets with parchment paper.

Put 1½ cups of the oats in a food processor and blitz until finely ground. Add the baking soda and salt, and pulse briefly to combine.

Place the coconut oil, honey, coconut sugar, tahini, eggs, and vanilla in a large bowl and beat well to combine. Tip in the cherries and the dried ingredients, and mix just enough to incorporate.

Using a large cookie scoop, place the mixture onto the prepared baking sheets; flatten slightly and leave a 2-inch (5 cm) space between to allow them to spread.

Bake for 12 minutes, until just starting to turn golden around the edges but still a little soft in the middle. Leave the cookies to cool on the baking sheets for 2 minutes, and then transfer to a wire rack to cool completely.

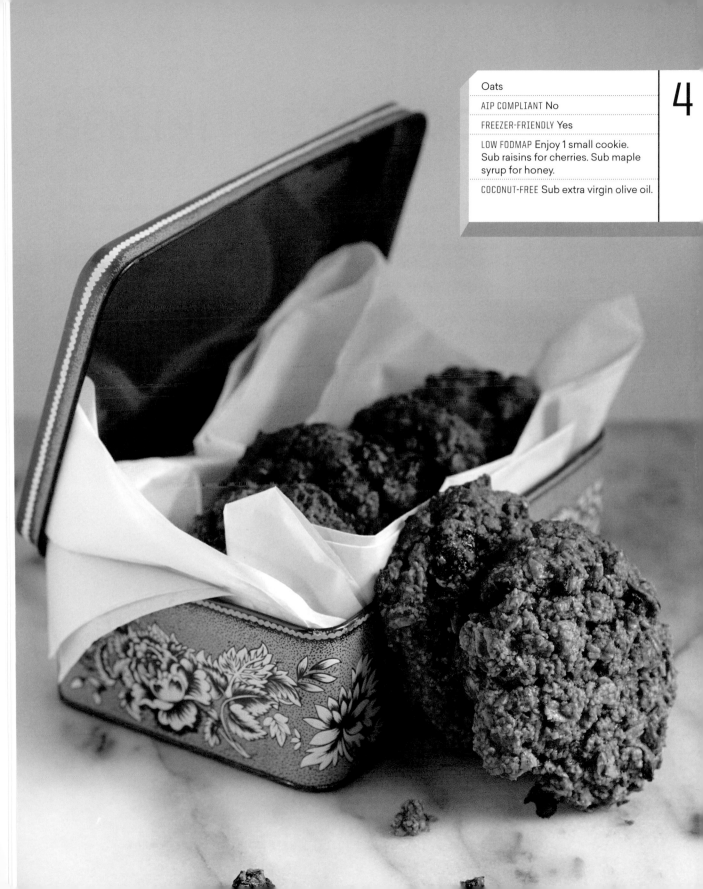

Oats

AIP COMPLIANT No

FREEZER-FRIENDLY Yes

LOW FODMAP Enjoy 1 small cookie. Sub raisins for cherries. Sub maple syrup for honey.

COCONUT-FREE Sub extra virgin olive oil.

4

INDEX

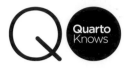
First Published in 2021 by Fair Winds Press, an imprint of The Quarto Group, 100 Cummings Center, Suite 265-D, Beverly, MA 01915, USA.
T (978) 282-9590 F (978) 283-2742 QuartoKnows.com

Fair Winds Press titles are also available at discount for retail, wholesale, promotional, and bulk purchase. For details, contact the Special Sales Manager by email at specialsales@quarto.com or by mail at The Quarto Group, Attn: Special Sales Manager, 100 Cummings Center, Suite 265-D, Beverly, MA 01915, USA.

25 24 23 22 21   1 2 3 4 5

ISBN: 978-1-59233-973-0

Digital edition published in 2021
eISBN: 978-1-63159-917-0

Library of Congress Cataloging-in-Publication Data available.

Design: Stacy Wakefield-Forte
Page Layout: Stacy Wakefield-Forte
Photography: Kate Jay and Jamie-Lee Fuoco page 203

Printed in China

The information in this book is for educational purposes *only. It is not intended to replace the advice of a physician or medical practitioner. Please see your health-care provider before beginning any new health program.*